SELF-INSTRUCTION
IN MEDICAL EDUCATION

SELF-INSTRUCTION
IN MEDICAL EDUCATION

Proceedings of the Second Rochester Conference, on
June 24-26, 1965

Jerome P. Lysaught and Hilliard Jason
Editors

THE ROCHESTER CLEARINGHOUSE
on Self-Instructional Materials for Health Care Facilities

 The University of Rochester

*To those many individuals
who have never lost sight
of the essence of learning
while meeting the many
other demands of the modern
medical school—the faculty
members listed in this volume
and their colleagues, many of
whom will be known only to and
through their students.*

W
18
R676p
1965

Printed in the United States of America.

Library of Congress Catalog Card Number: 67-28368

Preface

It was in June of 1965 that the Second Rochester Conference was held. By its title alone, there was demonstrated some indication of the rapid change that has taken place in medical education over a comparatively short period of time. In June of 1965, the First Rochester Conference was devoted to "Programmed Instruction in Medical Education." A year later, the conference was broadened to become, "Self-Instruction in Medical Education." The difference reflected is more than semantic. Many improvements had taken place in technology, frequently reflecting further insights into theory and application. Moreover, wiser and longer analysis of programmed instruction emphasized its tremendous properties as a process—properties far more important than its mere product in text or machine form as a learning program. This process promised to improve any instructional form to which it was applied, and most particularly any approaches through which the individual may work as a self-paced, self-evaluating learner. Self-instructional films, tapes, simulators, teaching computers and other advances, based firmly on the methodological foundation of programmed instruction, bade fair to provide increased flexibility and wider capability than the limited programmed texts that were initially introduced.

In the pages of this volume, medical educators and selected specialists from other fields analyze the developing state of the art and report detailed experience in the use of self-instructional materials. In comparison to the contents of the first proceedings, we find quite as many questions, but more answers in terms of documented efficiency, effectiveness, and capability of programmed learning in the medical curriculum. We see its extension into foreign schools, and its steady growth into more and more areas of clinical and preclinical instruction. We also can observe the enlargement of its process significance as *programmed tests, programmed lectures,* and *programmed patients* become more common terms in medical teaching—each one reflecting unique adaptations of the fundamental programming methodology.

The papers from the Conference have been slightly rearranged for publication in order that they might present the most logical development to the reader. Part I is an overview, a summary and analysis of research to date, and a speculative look at the impacts of self-instruction on the future medical school. Part II provides an answer to the perplexing question of how to select and evaluate a programmed sequence for the health field. Part III consists of a series of controlled research studies on effectiveness of self-instructional materials in medical education, and includes a study from England and one from Spain to demonstrate the cross-cultural implications of this instructional methodology. Part IV consists of less rigorous studies primarily aimed at exploring the practical curricular implications of new techniques and technologies. Part V deals with interesting extensions of the basic modality of programming, applying it to lectures, tests, and live simulators or "patients." Part VI is a summary and review paper that seeks to describe what has been learned and to suggest where the next steps ought to be directed.

It is regrettable that the limitations of physical publication in book form prevent our being able to convey the discussions that took place in the small group sessions scheduled at intervals throughout the course of the Conference. I would like to thank, however, the individuals who served as resource people for these groups, particularly those who filled this role we asked of them and, in so doing, gave up an opportunity to prepare a formal paper for publication. They include: John W. Blyth, Vice President, Argyle Publishing Company; Thomas Hale Ham, Director, Division of Research in Medical Education, Western Reserve University School of Medicine; and Leon Summit, then Editor of Pfizer *Spectrum*. Each one of these persons contributed generously and unselfishly of his time and talent.

To the members of the conference committee from the faculty of the University of Rochester, I would like to express sincere gratitude. Mrs. Josephine Craytor of the Department of Nursing, Charles D. Sherman, Jr. of the Department of Surgery, and Clarence M. Williams of the College of Education contributed to the planning and carrying out of the program with professional dispatch.

To the Editorial Staff of Pfizer *Spectrum* who were instrumental in the publication of the first proceedings, and who aided us in the work on this second volume out of personal friendship and belief in its importance, I can only say that our appreciation knows no limits. Leon Summit, Julian Becker, Glenda Hight, and their co-workers have gone far beyond the call of duty long after their formal connection to the project through their firm was dissolved.

Thanks also to Mrs. Jeannine Korman, Mrs. Virginia Mulford, Mrs. Dorothy Johnson, and Miss Judy Dorman who worked without complaint on the many typings and revisions; to Miss Sydney Sutherland who read and proofed the manuscript; to Jack Spring and Donald Haefele who worked on the coordination and presentation of the Conference; and to our many associates in the College of Education and the School of Medicine and Dentistry who extended themselves to aid us in this undertaking.

Within the pages of this volume, you will find the work and contributions of nearly thirty authors and co-authors. In order to blend their many styles into one balanced manuscript, the editors have sometimes taken liberty with their words and phrases, but never with their ideas or their positions. For that which is contained in these papers that is useful and developmental, credit must go to the authors. For errors of either omission or commission, the editors accept full responsibility.

It has been in many respects a labor of love to work with these proceedings. Those of you who find them worthwhile and stimulating may wish to avail yourselves of the services of our Clearinghouse on Self-Instructional Materials for Health Care Facilities which offers a number of aids, including a periodic bulletin which is sent without charge, by means of an educational grant from the Kellogg Foundation through the Hospital Research and Educational Trust.

JEROME P. LYSAUGHT
Coordinator,
Rochester Clearinghouse

Rochester, New York
April 1, 1967

Contents

Part IV: Curricular Applications of Self-Instruction

Part V: Extensions of the Programming Process

Part VI: Summary and Perspective

Part I

A Framework for Viewing Self-Instruction

In the introductory paper, McKee raises anew the enduring questions of professional education and challenges the new methodologies and technologies of self-instruction to contribute to their solution. Lysaught summarizes the present state of the art and proposes a set of general statements that seem to follow from research and experimentation. Jason projects these findings into their logical implications for the medical school of the future, its curriculum, and its teaching practices.

A Focus and a Change

FRANK W. McKEE, M.D.*

IT IS MY PRIVILEGE to welcome you today on behalf of our students and faculty to this second Rochester Conference on Self-Instruction in Medical Education. Having been involved as a pathologist in some rather basic areas of medical education at all levels—the medical student, the postgraduate student, and the practitioner—for something over twenty years, I cannot but commend the imagination and enterprise that are being exerted in this interesting development. Certainly, in our era of increasing research and burgeoning printed material, with a need to offer greater areas of information and developed knowledge to so many thirsting people—both lay and professional—it is profoundly important to devise new methods and approaches for the promulgation of basic and useful data so that it can be mastered effectively and productively.

Among the first examples of self-instruction that come to my mind, is the story, perhaps apocryphal, of the boy Abraham Lincoln, by the light of the fireplace, copying words and numbers from a borrowed book, writing with a piece of charcoal on a wooden shovel, and then scraping the surface clear to start again. The real message, to me, of this story of a school boy working away without pencil and paper, is the industry and dedication portrayed by a youngster who desperately wanted to learn, and do, and apply. I can only presume that he was aware his goals and ambitions extended beyond the im-

*Then Acting Dean, now Associate Dean and Professor of Pathology, University of Rochester School of Medicine and Dentistry.

mediate urge to learn. However this may have been, a general opportunity for self-instruction is now a fact of life in a variety of educational fields, and offers additional impetus within the reach of many people for self-improvement and the acquisition of increasing information.

Even so, I think it is important for me to inject a note of caution against too great a dependence on, or enthusiasm for, this particular *modus operandi* as anything but an adjunct to the educational process, particularly as it relates to medical education. There are several reasons for this; I will cite but three which are particularly relevant in the context of physician training, although they may have a general bearing on other fields of education.

First there is the teacher-student relationship, which is probably more important in medical education than in any other profession.

There are two broad faces to medicine: the science and the art. I submit that in the enlargement and ascendancy of the former, and the comparative shrinkage and regression of the latter, lie many of the major problems confronting the profession today. At a precommencement talk to our now newest graduates, I commented as follows: If one looks for the message for the physician of today, it comes down to the relatively simple question of just what is his engagement with the patients whose lives are entrusted to him. Human society is so constituted that it needs moral and spiritual support, along with synthetic blood vessels, transplanted organs, and the latest information, drug or technique. Whether a patient is moderately ill, or facing death, or "just a hypochondriac," the strength and tradition of medicine has been that it provides support, comfort and understanding, and seeks a rapport far beyond that of any other profession with its clientele.

And while the need for this part of medicine—the so-called art— is easily accepted intellectually by the professionally unsophisticated and naive premedical student as he prepares to engage himself in his chosen career, the art itself is dreadfully hard to teach in medical school; for it relies on the character and integrity of the individual student, drawn out and tempered by his contacts with, and the character of, his teachers, fellow students and patients. The intellect of the medical graduate and seasoned physician will rarely be a matter of concern; his ability to solve the problems of diagnosis and treatment in a world of increasing paramedical handmaidens and prepackaged panaceas will rarely cause trouble. But his relationships with patients and colleagues, which are many times the turning point in true medical success, will always be the great unknown, and will become the fulcrum on which success and failure teeter back and forth.

Is this achieved by being "on guard"? Isn't it rather achieved by developing qualities or attitudes like those described in the preceding phrases? Therefore, one must ever seek to fortify his personal enthusiasm, his devotion to his fellow man and his profession, and his constant careful distinction between right and wrong, until the strength of these qualities is at least equal to that of his medical knowledge in the pursuit of a high standard of professional integrity and purpose.

The need for close relationship between teacher and student in achieving the foundation for this necessary attitude is covered in a cogent statement by George W. Corner, our respected first professor of anatomy. Dr. Corner has said,

> "The ideal association between teacher and student can be summed up in one principle, which is that students learn the medical sciences and clinical medicine not from didactic teaching, but by working at science and medicine as members of the laboratories and clinics; standing side by side with experienced men; listening in the lecture room not to mere repetitious pedagogues, but to trained minds wrestling with current problems; doing as nearly as possible what their teachers are doing; [and] in the later years . . . carrying on their own shoulders as much of the hospital's responsibilities as can possibly be given them."

We must be sure, in a profession which is dependent on example and model as well as the accumulation of knowledge, that we erect no formidable interference or barrier to the basic premises on which so much of the success of the physician rests.

A second point in medical education requiring some caution is a recognition that the "facts" are ever-changing. When I was in medical school some twenty odd years ago, the drug companies were just beginning to issue the categorical booklets, replete with clear exposition and colored illustration, of a wide variety of diseases, systems, organs, processes and procedures. I can remember sending off a number of 1¢ post cards, with some fiscal trepidation, to secure this bounty. Today, I look at some of these now historical references and find considerable change in concept and so-called fact. While history is well served in such review, medical knowledge, as we accept it today, is not. Therefore, the overemphasis on the engagement of the student and the physician with the detail and minutiae of present-day information, and the learning thereof, may actually be an overemphasis on current opinion, which is subject to change and vulnerable to serious error, as concepts and principles change. This may not be true in certain fundamental areas, such as gross anatomy, but I point out that one should recognize the evanescence and mutability of information and even knowledge.

The teacher should concern himself with the essence of education. This essence is the development in the student of the ability to think and reason, rather than to encumber himself with a surfeit of detailed theory and trivia or opinion that tomorrow may be outdated, passé and valueless, or superseded by something more plausible, more applicable, or again only temporarily successful. The care and feeding of the mind as a functional, reasoning mechanism is the goal of the true educative process.

The third point I would stress is that there is considerable difference between knowledge and wisdom. As William Cowper has said, "Knowledge and wisdom, far from being one, have oft-times no connection. Knowledge dwells in heads replete with thoughts of other men; wisdom in minds attentive to their own. Knowledge is proud that he knows so much. Wisdom is humble that he knows no more."

In medical education and its application, it is wisdom that we hope our graduates will possess and develop—so that the blending of accumulated knowledge and experience will enable a wide range of appropriate success, rather than encourage a contrary narrowness and inhibition, resulting in either misapplication of knowledge or inability to use it at all. Another factor—information—overwhelms us these days, particularly in our medical journals and other publications. In spite of all sorts of devices and machinery to categorize and collate, we may never recover from this avalanche of information, the significance of which can hardly be judged until it is assimilated and stands some test of application. Information requires human cerebral processing before it can qualify as knowledge, and needs the tempering fires of experience to rework and expand it into the final gem of wisdom.

So I leave with you these three fundamental theses which are so major a part of medical education—(1) the necessity of the intimate teacher-student relationship; (2) the primary emphasis on training the mind to deal with innovation, association and change in the face of the instability and constant metamorphosis of medical information; and (3) the final goal of the competent, compassionate, involved physician, who recognizes patients as human beings in need of his skills and the wisdom of his effort, rather than the stultified practitioner, confused, and essentially paralyzed by an overstock of unmanageable, fragmented and therefore useless information, and handicapped by an understock of human understanding and compassion.

The role of self-instruction in medical education, particularly at the undergraduate level, I believe, is presently not solidly defined, and we eagerly wait for it to prove its ultimate value as a blessed and respected adjunct, or to earn its eventual castigation as a meddlesome deterrent, to the education—in its full meaning—of the physician. Self-instruction in selected phases of the science of medicine has exciting possibilities; but it must neither be overdone in this area nor oppress or depress the concomitant development of the art of medicine—an area where it may have little place.

I hope you will enjoy your time with us here in Rochester, and that your meetings will be profitable to yourselves, to your institutions, and to the cause of medical education—the training of physicians—which, in these times, cannot have too many adherents and participants.

EDITORIAL DATAGRAM:

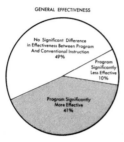

Figure 1. Comparison of Programmed and Conventional Instruction on General Effectiveness (Achievement + Efficiency).

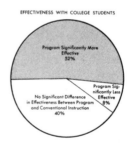

Figure 2. Comparison of Programmed and Conventional Instruction on General Effectiveness with College Students Only.

Summary Results of Multiple Studies on Programmed Instruction. For a discussion see the *Bulletin of the Clearinghouse on Self-Instructional Materials for Health Care Facilities,* Vol. 1, No. 2, July, 1966.

What We See Today

JEROME P. LYSAUGHT, Ed.D.*

WE ARE MEETING today on almost the anniversary of the first conference to have been devoted to the exclusive examination of programmed, self-instructional materials in medical education. In an age in which we have become rather comfortably adjusted to the fact that things happen rapidly and dramatically, we are perhaps too prone to accept the manifestations of these changes without remembering the expenditure of energy and effort that preceded the accomplishment.

It may not be amiss to recall briefly the history of instructional program development in medical education. In 1958, the first "learning program" was administered to undergraduate students in psychology at Harvard. In 1961, the Dartmouth Medical School Project in self-instruction came into being. This project in the following year was using the first recorded medical program, a sequence in the field of parasitology. In 1963, this program, in turn, became the first commercially published self-instructional medical program. By June of 1965, there were more than 25 available teaching programs that could be utilized by medical educators. And, by an inspection of publishers' announcement lists, it is anticipated that the present rate of growth will be maintained over the next two or three years at least.

The growth in availability of programs has been accompanied by a marked growth in their use, particularly in the medical colleges of

*Associate Professor of Education and Research Associate in Medical Education, The University of Rochester College of Education and School of Medicine and Dentistry.

this country. A survey of medical schools in 1964[1] revealed that 17 per cent of these institutions were using programmed materials, and almost 40 per cent had one or more faculty members actively engaged in a research or development project in this area. While no comparable figures are available for 1965, there is strong indication that the growth in use has been considerable. More than two thirds of the country's medical colleges have indicated that they are using the Pfizer allergy program as an instructional device.[2] This alone would be a four-fold increase in the number of institutions using self-instructional sequences. It likely represents only a base line of utilization, since it is reasonable to presume that some schools not using this particular program have found other self-instructional units useful.

Similarly, the number of institutions engaged in research on, or development of, self-instructional materials seems to be growing— although this is largely a subjective impression based on our correspondence through the Rochester Clearinghouse. In addition, the American experience in self-instruction for medical education is being examined closely and is beginning to be applied in medical schools around the world.

While much has happened swiftly, we are now at a point where we can propose some initial generalizations that seem to be supported both by research evidence and practical experience. In the remainder of this paper, I will discuss briefly several of these findings.

1. Programs are effective instructional devices.

Study after study has contributed to our certainty that self-instructional programs are effective with students. In the earliest study at the Dartmouth Medical School, Green, Weiss, and Nice[3] reported that students using an instructional program in parasitology attained significantly higher scores on achievement tests than did matched students taught by the lecture method.

In a larger research project at the University of Illinois College of Medicine,[4] three separate studies indicated that the programmed materials were at least as effective—and in a number of cases more effective—than lectures and conventional classroom presentations. Interestingly enough, these findings seem to have upset rather than to have favorably impressed the principal investigator, who concluded that "it would be pointless to deny that the findings were disappointing." I am not certain what findings were anticipated, but

I find it astonishing to be unhappy with the evidence that we can do at least as well with an explicit teaching model as we can with conventional instruction.

Eaton and his associates[5] have similarly reported on the use of self-instructional programmed units in basic psychopathology. Again, the "program" students exceeded their "control group" peers in achievement—although not with statistical significance.

While each of the three studies mentioned above used the traditional control group design, there have been a number of studies aimed at determining the effectiveness of self-instructional programs in a definitive, absolute way, without reference to the comparable achievement of students taught by lecture or by other conventional methods.

Brooke and Reynolds have described their work in developing material in amebiasis.[6] Their desired goal was to obtain for each student a score of 100 per cent on a final test of achievement. Other kinds of teaching had previously failed to meet such a criterion. After completion of the field testing of the program, they found that their primary trainee population groups ranged from 87 per cent to 100 per cent on the post-test median scores. Moreover, an analysis of errors indicated specific areas in which improvement could be made in the program to further enhance achievement.

In similar fashion, Rondell, Geis and Zinn[7] have reported the use of a program, *Diffusion and Osmosis,* that produced a class mean of 93 per cent on the post-test, with students from the bottom quintile of the class achieving 90 per cent scores.

2. Programs are efficient instructional devices.

Coupled with the concern for effectiveness in medical education is the companion consideration of efficiency—in the time required of both students and teachers. With so much to learn, and such precious little time available, there is a need to examine the efficiency of self-instructional programs.

Green, Weiss, and Nice[3] report a high factor of efficiency. Computation of an efficiency index for each participating student in their research on the parasitology program indicated that the program students learned far more efficiently than did their control comparisons. This difference between the two groups was significant at the .01 level.

In the study on a program in body fluid metabolism at the University of Illinois College of Medicine,[4] it was found that the students using programs at three schools not only achieved more in terms of post-test scores, but took less time to do so. In two of the three schools, this difference was statistically significant at the .05 level. Despite the restrained way in which the findings are reported, it would be far from hazardous to suggest that a study of total effectiveness which used both achievement and efficiency factors would almost inevitably establish the superiority of the program, with statistical significance.

In their study on self-instruction in psychopathology, Eaton and his associates[5] suggest that the program was more efficient than other instruction even though the experimental situation required the use of slides rather than programmed texts, thus reducing the efficiency that potentially could have been obtained.

Efficiency, however, is measured not only in terms of the average time expenditure of a class, but also by the utilization of each individual's learning time. As in studies of achievement, there are some studies of efficiency of learning in absolute terms, rather than in terms of comparison with a control or "conventional" group.

One of these has been reported in connection with the study of *Allergy and Hypersensitivity*.[2] On the basis of some 5,500 returns it is possible to report that the average time required to complete the program was approximately 5 hours, with perhaps two thirds of the users completing the material in the range from 4 to 6 hours. There were a number of individuals who took 2 hours or less to complete the program; with the provision in the self-instructional process for them to move at their optimum rate, they conserved their time. Some users, however, reported taking over 20 hours to complete the same sequence. This 10x factor of difference in learning time is not surprising to the educational psychologist. It may, however, be surprising to some lecturers. In any event, the program permitted instructional adaptation to the extremes of individual needs. It could even be argued, of course, that provision of such variable periods for learning is an example of sheer efficiency if the alternative is that the student would otherwise not have learned, or not have learned to a sufficient degree.

Another example of a study of absolute efficiency is to be found in the report of Brooke and Reynolds.[6] Their criterion of absolute achievement was accompanied by an actual reduction in required learning time.

3. Programs are accepted by the learners.

In examining the results of program utilization, it is worth noting that student reaction to self-instructional methods has generally been quite positive.

The Dartmouth Study[3] indicated that the combination of small steps and reinforcement utilized within the program contributed not only to efficiency of student handling, but also to improved classroom performance on the part of many students who could now take part in discussions and problem-solving exercises more meaningfully. These students "liked" the program for its demonstrated helpfulness.

The Nebraska study[5] reported that the "experimental group expressed a definite preference for programmed instruction rather than lectures and textbook assignments."

In the survey on *Allergy and Hypersensitivity*[2] a sub-sample of medical students provides us with some interesting information on their reactions to the self-instructional process. Two hundred students from a variety of medical schools were asked this question: "In comparison with the same amount of time spent on other forms of educational reading matter or instruction, do you find this type review of more, equal, or less value?" Seventy-seven per cent of the students indicated they felt the program to be of more value; 20 per cent replied that it was of equal value; less than 2 per cent felt it to be of less value. This reaction is statistically significant at well beyond the .001 level.

When asked whether they would like to receive other programs in different subject matter areas, 100 per cent of the respondents said "yes." (This included those individuals who had felt programs to be of "less" value. At the very least, this finding indicates commendable willingness of the medical student to reserve final judgment.)

Two studies have reported results that differ in part from the findings discussed so far. In a pilot study on the use of self-instructional materials in hematology,[8] it was found that all students tended to achieve well using the individual study materials. However, these who were most critical of the material actually achieved more than those who were most favorably inclined toward the process. This would seem to argue against too easy an assertion of a Hawthorne effect, and perhaps suggests that thoughtful criticism by students may contribute to future improvements in the self-instructional process.

At the University of Oklahoma Medical Center[9] residents in psychiatry demonstrated remarkable avoidance behavior toward the use of a teaching machine program. Since only one of the thirteen residents actually completed the program, it may be fair to suggest that self-instruction was not the real issue. The program may simply have brought to a head a number of matters related to training in that department.

In any event, although the overwhelming reaction of students is favorable, no panacea is claimed, and negative findings deserve further study and analysis.

4. Programs have produced other positive learning results.

The report of the hematology study[8] concluded with the observation that "the students did accept the added responsibility for their own learning." Also, the students "achieved significantly higher on the problem-solving section of the examination," which required them to apply cognitive learning to a simulated case.

Christensen[10] has emphasized the utility of programmed sequences for providing individualized remedial instruction, in anticipation of a new course, that permits a student to make up deficiencies which would otherwise put him at a disadvantage in comparison with his classmates.

Finally, the Dartmouth Project[3] reported that the program had succeeded in constructing for the students a guide to desired learning objectives which permitted them to discriminate validly between those things which they had to learn and those things which would be "nice" to learn.

5. Programs have a wide variety of curricular uses.

In terms of the over-all medical school curriculum, it is clear that the approximately 25 programmed sequences available today can provide only a beginning. It should be noted, however, that there is already a fair distribution of programs among preclinical and clinical subjects, among both general and specialized fields of information.

It should be recognized that many of the large—and increasing—number of academic programs in fields related to medicine will have their impact on medical teaching. For example, medical colleges have already[11] reported the use under certain circumstances of programs in chemistry, biology, statistics, and psychology. It is probable that self-instructional materials in a variety of other fields will prove helpful as either review, remedial, or enrichment texts.

It can also be pointed out that most of the available sequences in medicine are short units based on neatly circumscribed objectives. This is seen by Sanazaro[12] and others as providing a maximum of flexibility while maintaining excellence. A short sequence on *pH and Dissociation,* for example, will permit use of the program in varying ways by different schools; one school may use it, for example, in the first semester of the first year; a second school may use it in the second semester; and a third may require its successful completion before classes begin. Under differing circumstances, it may be used for initial instruction, for review, and possibly for remedial purposes. It can be easily moved within the semester sequence to fit the purposes of an individual instructor.

All these considerations can be summed up in the concept that the curriculum becomes unfrozen as a greater number of proven alternatives become available for teaching. In addition, many of these instructional materials will have value for continuing education. While a conventional text may not intrigue a practitioner into exploring a subject, he may be quite attracted by a rich variety of programs with their more limited and clearly discernible objectives. Preliminary research evidence already available indicates that this is so.[2]

6. Programs have a rich taxonomy of learning outcomes.

Much of the criticism of early programs in academic fields turned on the point that they were for "rote" subjects and drill kinds of learning. There is more than a little truth in this observation; there were perhaps 20 programs in elementary algebra before we had the first commercial program in the social sciences.

It is to the credit of the early investigators of programming in medicine that they moved rather rapidly beyond the concrete levels of cognitive learning to the more abstract areas of understanding, generalization, and synthesis. The teaching of electrocardiography, for example, involves a complex combination of cognitive and motor skills. In a different way, the teaching of allergy involves the handling of competitive theories and outright disagreements. The authors of these programs have displayed a willingness and a capacity to do more in programming than to rest content with the basic elucidation of low-order facts.

The successful development by Wilds[13] of programmed materials in the judgmental areas of diagnosis and patient management is an even more illustrative example of the implications of self-instructional techniques for the future. Among the available programs, and those known to be under development, can be found examples of the entire learning taxonomy from both the cognitive and affective domains[14,15]. This suggests that the principal limitation on "what may be programmed" will be the imagination of the programmer himself.

7. Programs have growing process significance for education.

In addition to the effect that is registered by their teaching performance, there are some benefits of the research on, and development of, self-instructional programs that may be of even more significance to the curriculum.

There is nothing unique in the requirements that the development of a program places on an instructor. What is unique is that this occurs in such an explicit way that we cannot slight aspects of the teaching-learning situation which we have so long accepted in principle, but have so infrequently carried out in practice.

For example, the programming process requires that we examine the student, individually and collectively. Sanazaro[12] has pointed out that there are rather wide ranges of ability among medical students, yet we seldom acknowledge the fact that textbooks should presumably have differential effects upon these different learners. In the Dartmouth Project[3] it was found that there were differential effects on the bottom fifth of the learners, and in a later report[16] it was shown that these differences were increased when the program was tried in other medical schools. These differences are real; we ignore them only at our own peril—or that of our students. An objective evaluation of student response to self-instructional materials, however, provides us with a clearer guide toward structuring alternative approaches that will be equally successful over a broader range of learner differences.

The increased emphasis on the objectives of instruction is beginning to make its impact felt. Sherman and his colleagues[17] have reported the insights they obtained when they attempted to answer the seemingly simple question, "What should a medical student know about cancer of the breast?" Consider your own answer to that question in terms of what a student could do to demonstrate his satisfactory attainment of minimum competence.

There is a classic quality in the study by Pierce,[9] who discovered that the explicit nature of the programming process exposed the existence of semantic disagreements and misunderstandings among faculty members who had worked in daily communication with each other over a long period of time. They learned they simply could not agree on the definitions of a large number of basic terms that each was using frequently in his professional activities.

The programming process and its curricular effects do not stop at the boundary line of the program itself. We have reports from Roe[18] and others[19] that the teacher who has done some programming changes his own behavior as a result of what he himself learns from the experience. There are also two instances[20,21] in which a self-instructional program has been successfully rendered into a discursive text—while at the same time there is ample evidence that the reverse process is generally unsuccessful. These findings would indicate that the explicit techniques required to construct a good program are at least as important to its eventual success as any incidental factors involving student response mechanisms and methods of presenting material.

Finally, as we will see in other reports in this volume, the theory of programming is having important effects on testing, large-group instruction, and other media such as teaching films.

8. Programs have curricular applications beyond the medical college.

If a new approach is effective, we can generally predict that it will come to bear on more objects than those which were expected to be its primary targets. As already suggested, academic programs in various specialty fields will likely find useful applications in the medical college. The reverse will undoubtedly be equally true. We have also mentioned the use of medical school material in continuing education, and early research on the use of programmed materials with practitioners has been quite encouraging.

Research studies in other areas also have important implications for future work in medical education. There is broadening use of programs for the paramedical field. Some materials initially intended for medical students, with appropriate modification, have been successfully adapted to the training of nurses, technicians, and semiprofessional employees. There is evidence that the application of programming principles to instruction can increase the learning achievement of paramedical personnel and, at the same time, reduce the wide variation in terminal performance that often is found today.[23]

There is even some research directed at the use of self-instructional materials with the non-professional employees of medical centers and hospitals.[24] While this is only very indirectly an offshoot of developmental work in medical education, it is of great importance for the future role of the doctor. Since even the most capable practitioner must rely from time to time on the performance of many "unskilled," a growth in their ability to perform well is inevitably to his advantage.

A last example of this broadening range of curricular applications is the increasing number of studies on the teaching of patient self-care.[25] This has significance for two reasons. First, any increase in learning effectiveness and efficiency in this area will aid both the patient and the physician. Second, programs may help the physician to provide for the very wide range of patient instruction which is frequently necessary, but for which he is not specifically trained. It is encouraging that the reaction of patients has been most positive to early trials of such materials.[25]

Summary

Let me summarize for you briefly the generalizations that seem to follow from the first four years of research and utilization of self-instructional materials in medical education:

1. Learning programs are effective instructional devices.

2. Learning programs are efficient instructional devices.

3. Programs have been positively received by medical students and practitioners.

4. Learning programs have contributed to beneficial results in terms of increased student responsibility and improved learning habits.

5. Programs offer a wide variety of curricular uses.

6. Programs represent a wide range of learning outcomes from rote learning to complex cognitive levels.

7. Apart from the value of the programs themselves, the process of programming offers new approaches to the improvement

of teaching and learning.

8. Programs have demonstrated curricular applications beyond the medical college.

There is still much research to be done. More exploration of the curricular implications of self-instruction is needed. To the sophisticated viewer of research, much of what has been done to date may appear oversimplified, and even trite. He may say that we have done enough of the comparative studies, and enough of the exploratory field trials, and that some important dimensions are still untouched. Let me reply in the words of Sam Johnson, "When it shall be found that much is omitted, let it not be forgotten that much likewise is performed."

As we consider the record of research on self-instruction in medical education, let us remember that it is of only four years' duration, and for a four year old it is amazingly well-developed and strong. Having said that, we must turn to the tasks that remain. The speakers who follow over the course of this conference will be reporting on many of these "next steps" which they have already undertaken.

References

1. Lysaught, J. P., Sherman, C. C., and Williams, C. M. "Utilization of Programmed Instruction in Medical Education." *J. Med. Educ.* 39:769-773 (September) 1964.

2. Lysaught, J. P. "Programmed Instruction for Medical Education: Learner Reactions to a Large Scale Use." *New Phys.* 14:156-160 (June) 1965.

3. Green, E. J., Weiss, R. J., and Nice, P. O. "Experimental Use of a Programmed Text in a Medical School Course." *J. Med. Educ.* 37:767-775 (August) 1962.

4. Miller, G. E. "Report to the Faculty, 1963-1964. University of Illinois, College of Medicine, Office of Research in Medical Education." Offset. pp 77-80.

5. Eaton, M. T., Strough, L. C., and Muffly, R. B. "Programmed Instruction in Basic Psychopathology." *J. Med. Educ.* 39:36-89 (January) 1964.

6. Brooke, M. M., and Reynolds, R. L. "Preliminary Evaluation of a Program: 'Amebiasis—Laboratory Diagnosis,'" in Lysaught, J. P. (ed.) *Programmed Instruction in Medical Education*. Rochester, N. Y.: The University of Rochester, 1965.

7. Rondell, P. A., Geis, G. L., and Zinn, K. L. "A Program in Diffusion and Osmosis: An Evaluation," in Lysaught, J. P. (ed.) *Programmed Instruction in Medical Education*. Rochester, N. Y.: The University of Rochester, 1965.

8. Harris, J. W., Horrigan, D. L., Ginther, J. R. and Ham, T. H. "Pilot Study in Teaching Hematology, with emphasis on Self-Education by the Students." *J. Med. Educ.* 37:719-736 (August) 1962.

9. Pierce, C. M., Pishkin, V., and Mathis, J. L. "Some Problems in Developing a Psychiatric Program," in Lysaught, J. P. (ed.) *Programmed Instruction in Medical Education.* Rochester, N. Y.: The University of Rochester, 1965.

10. Christensen, H. N. "The Identification of Special Topics for Teaching by Short 'Plug-In' Programs," in Lysaught, J. P. (ed.) *Programmed Instruction in Medical Education.* Rochester, N. Y.: The University of Rochester, 1965.

11. Lysaught, J. P. "Self-Instructional Medical Programs: A Survey." *New Phys.* 13:101-107. (April) 1964.

12. Sanazaro, P. "Applications of Programming in Medical Education," in Lysaught, J. P. (ed.) *Programmed Instruction in Medical Education.* Rochester, N. Y.: The University of Rochester, 1965.

13. Wilds, P. L. "Programmed Instruction as a Method of Teaching Clinical Problem-Solving," in Lysaught, J. P. (ed.) *Programmed Instruction in Medical Education.* Rochester, N. Y.: The University of Rochester, 1965.

14. Bloom, B. S., *et al. Taxonomy of Educational Objectives.* Handbook I: The Cognitive Domain. New York: Longmans, Green, 1956.

15. Krathwohl, D. R., *et al. Taxonomy of Educational Objectives.* Handbook II: The Affective Domain. New York: McKay, 1964.

16. Nice, P. O., *et al. Medical Parasitology.* New York: Appleton-Century-Crofts, 1963.

17. Sherman, C. D., Jr., Lysaught, J. P., and Williams, C. M. "Problems in Developing Concepts and Goals in Programmed Instruction," in Lysaught, J. P. (ed.) *Programmed Instruction in Medical Education.* Rochester, N. Y.: The University of Rochester, 1965.

18. Roe, A., *et al.* "Automated Teaching Methods Using Linear Programs." Report No. 60-105, Dept. of Engineering, Univ. of California at Los Angeles, December, 1960.

19. Lysaught, J. P. "The Effects of the Preparation and Utilization of Automated Teaching on the Classroom Teacher," in Roucek, J. S. (ed.) *Automated Teaching.* New York: Philosophical Library, 1965.

20. Bernstein, L. M., Allender, J., and Miller, G. E. "Teaching Fundamental Concepts of Renal Physiology Using Programmed Materials." Paper delivered at the Rochester Conference on Programmed Instruction in Medical Education, 1964.

21. Summit, Leon. "Team Programming in Medical Instruction," in Lysaught, J. P. (ed.) *Programmed Instruction in Medical Education.* Rochester, N. Y.: The University of Rochester, 1965.

22. Spiegel, A. D. "Evaluation of an Automated Teaching Machine Program for Continuing Education of Physicians." *Mass. Gen. Pract. News.* 13:12-14 (March) 1964.

23. Craytor, J. K. and Lysaught, J. P. "Programmed Instruction in Nursing Education: A Trial Use." *Nursing Research.* 13:323-326 (Fall) 1964.

24. Carter, E. J., Moore, A. N., and Gregory, C. L. "Can Teaching Machines Help in Training Employees?" *Journal of the American Dietetic Association.* 44:271-276 (April) 1964.

25. Nickerson, H. H. "A Teaching Machine for Diabetic Patients." *The Journal of the Maine Medical Association.* November, 1963.

EDITORIAL DATAGRAM:

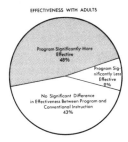

EFFECTIVENESS WITH ADULTS

Program Significantly More Effective
48%

Program Significantly Less Effective
9%

No Significant Difference in Effectiveness Between Program and Conventional Instruction
43%

Figure 3. Comparison of Programmed and Conventional Instruction on General Effectiveness with Adult Learners Only.

Summary Results of Multiple Studies on Adult Learning Programs. For a discussion see the *Bulletin of the Clearinghouse on Self-Instructional Materials for Health Care Facilities,* Vol. 1, No. 2, July, 1966.

A Glimpse of Tomorrow

HILLIARD JASON, M.D., Ed.D.*

MAY I INVITE YOU to join me in a brief, rather fanciful journey into the hazy and dimly lighted world of another time in another place. Our travels will take us to a land which does not have a counterpart in our present or past experience. In fact, to appreciate the language and customs of this land's inhabitants, we must temporarily put aside most of our usual expectations. Suspend, if you will, all recollection of classrooms, examinations and other familiar landmarks, and join Robert Smith, who has recently submitted his application and is going for his admission interviews to Metropolitan University School of Medicine.

It is worth noting, in passing, that Smith's premedical counselor, in consultation with the Applicant's Advisory Office of the Association of American Medical Colleges, had particularly recommended Metropolitan University because of Dr. Martin, the physiologist, with whom Smith might continue the work he has begun in relating the respiratory mechanisms of the salamander to devices for long-term human underwater living. The faculty at Metropolitan characteristically seek candidates with capabilities in an area closely related to the interests of one of their staff members. This stems from their belief that closely supervised, intensive investigative work provides a singularly satisfactory way to fulfill some central goals of their instructional program. In almost any area relevant to medicine, they

*Formerly, Associate in Medical Education and Assistant Professor of Psychiatry, The University of Rochester School of Medicine and Dentistry. Now, Director, Office of Medical Education Research and Development, and Associate Professor of Medicine and Education, Michigan State University Colleges of Human Medicine and of Education.

feel, work in depth enhances the student's capacity for independent, responsible scholarship, for skillful and critical data-gathering, for evaluation of evidence, and for developing the intellectual facilities and personal characteristics which are basic to both creative and deductive work.

All of these matters, the faculty contend, are indispensable to the pursuit of any of the many possible careers that will be available to Smith if he succeeds in becoming a physician. Indeed, so important are these attributes in their eyes, that if Smith is accepted, fully one third of his time may be spent in his chosen area of research.

Let us say that the selection committee is satisfied that Smith does meet their school's standards. With his acceptance, they send him some suggestions for strengthening a few areas which they have identified as minor weaknesses. In his final college months, his effort to extend his understanding of the ultramicroscopic investigation of chromosomal aberrations and to increase his competence with non-parametric statistics, will enable him to begin his work at the customary level at Metropolitan, and will permit him to proceed directly to his research program, avoiding the delay of remedial studies.

Some two months before enrollment, the "Program Coordination Office" of the medical school sends Smith a detailed outline of the goals of Phase I of the program, together with a comprehensive set of criteria by which he and the faculty will determine when he is ready to proceed to Phase II. He is told that the average student requires about six months for this first step, and that the range for most students is between three and nine months. He can see that he far surpasses the minimal criteria in respiratory physiology, but that he will need to devote considerable effort to compensate for his marginal background in auto-immune mechanisms and the characteristics of family organizational patterns. Actually, until now he hasn't given much thought to the importance of these matters in medicine. But, seeing the summary of goals for the entire medical course, he begins to conceive an early panoramic picture of the total task ahead and the rationale for the steps along the way. He can barely wait for this last free summer to end and for the work of becoming a physician to begin.

The first day of school is about the only time he can look around and see the student group that will be identified as the entering class of his year. While he will at times be working very closely with some of them, at other times he will join with students who entered before or after him. And, much of the time, he will be quite on his own.

One of the activities of this first day is a meeting with his advisory committee, those faculty members who will serve as his primary instructors throughout Phase I. These men, who represent a variety of medical disciplines, review with him the basic aim of this Phase, which is to help him gain a general conceptual understanding of disease processes. Some time ago the faculty at Metropolitan concluded that human learning is characterized by the process of going from the *general* to the *particular*. The soundest approach to medical study, they agreed, is to begin with a superficial overview of the simplest concepts of normal functioning and the forces which interfere with it. This approach provides a conceptual framework into which the students can later fit the details of medical knowledge. Only after Smith has acquired some beginning grasp of the general ways in which the integral human organism may be disrupted by, say, infectious, emotional or hereditary factors, will he begin to probe the depths of cell and organ structure and function and the specifics of human growth and development. His teachers have come to recognize, for example, that students are far more eager to learn about enzyme activity in glucose metabolism, and far more able to understand it, after, rather than before, they have some notion of the process of diabetes.

It is in this first phase of his work, Smith learns, that he will come to an appreciation of the key questions for which he will need answers, if he is to be a competent physician. Actually, some of his fellow students, from less advanced college backgrounds, find it paradoxical that the mark of success in Phase I will be that they will have learned to ask the *right questions* of their teachers. This becomes clearer to them, however, when they are presented, on color television tapes, the interviews and examinations of patients with certain general disorders, such as sickle-cell anemia, asthma or thyrotoxicosis. Not knowing the diagnosis, they have the task of requesting the *categories* of information needed to understand the patient's problem. The students discover that in the process they develop and refine their skills at being keen listeners and observers as well as critical thinkers. Many of them are surprised to learn how vital these operations are to the effective functioning of physicians, as well as how much can be learned about these matters once the task is clear and the supervision is sufficiently close and critical.

For some students, a primary goal of this Phase is that they learn to take major responsibility for their own learning. For most, this is not a problem; their prior schooling has all been characterized by reliance on their internal motivation, rather than on the imposition of artificial, external pressures.

Smith learns fairly quickly which member of his committee of instructors is likely to be most helpful with whatever problem he is having at any given time. At the start he notices he is unable to respond properly to the computerized self-evaluation quizzes because he has difficulty with some of the basic vocabulary in the video-taped interviews. Dr. Adams proves to be very skilled at helping him sort out the gaps in his understanding which have led to this vocabulary obstacle. Once this is overcome, Smith moves along smoothly for a short time, until the computer tabulations of his self-examination results show a fairly consistent failure to notice the surface markings of various disorders in the patients he is studying. He is steered to Dr. Bowen, who has organized a small group of students in similar need of assistance to sharpen their observational skills. They are soon "seeing" considerably more in most interpersonal settings, having learned to observe more critically. The exams next expose Smith's difficulty in gleaning much useful information from listening to patient histories. Smith is pleased to discover how much more he can "hear" as he becomes an increasingly skilled listener.

Toward the end of his second month of school, it becomes clear to both Smith and his committee that he has sufficient command of the basic tools to begin sinking his teeth into the substance of Phase I.

Now he is ready to gain some understanding of health and disease: of the similarities and differences between the child with a broken arm and the child whose pet dog was just killed; of the problems related to helping the unconscious accident victim, and the problems of the wife of the dying cancer patient. As he progresses through the more advanced aspects of Phase I, Smith notices how both his interests and activities are shading into the content of Phase II. In beginning to understand normal functioning and disease patterns he has become increasingly curious about the mechanisms and structures which are their basis.

During these last weeks of convincing both himself and his committee that he can meet and surpass all the criterion measures of

Phase I, he is beginning to browse in the Educational Resource Center for some introductory self-instructional materials on immunologic factors in organ transplants. He even finds a few hours now and then to go to his laboratory to begin practicing the methods and techniques he will need so that he can study Interferon production after adrenal transplantation as one of his projects in Phase II.

The ending of Phase I is quite inauspicious. The process of learning has been so interwoven with the process of self-testing that Smith and his committee have full documentation that he has indeed fulfilled all the didactic goals of this phase. Also, the committee members and Dr. Martin have had ample opportunity to assure themselves of Smith's fulfillment of their non-didactic expectations: of his integrity, dedication, and capacity both to assume responsibility and to take initiative. These are all of critical concern to the faculty, who recognize that it is in the early years of medical school that deficiencies in these areas must be identified. If remedial efforts are necessary, or if, in an extreme case, it is prudent to divert the student from further study of medicine, now is the time for appropriate action—for soon will come direct responsibility for patients, and hence, the very power of life and death.

Smith is delighted to find that Phase II is even more challenging and rewarding than Phase I. Now comes the privilege of delving to the heart of the mysteries of life. In the process of probing into the very essence of the diseases he is seeking to understand, he is coming to know much about the remarkably functional and endlessly fascinating intricacies of the physical and chemical structures of the human body, and about how they are tied together by interdependent and cross-connected systems which are complex beyond belief.

As he works with his Phase II committee, Smith finds himself using them differently from his Phase I committee. Instead of looking to them for assistance in finding the cause of his failure to perceive or identify certain issues he is now asking them to guide him in the process of unscrambling highly complex problems and searching for plausible solutions. Along the way, Smith finds he has many new laboratory techniques to master, and technical skills to perfect. The self-instructional cartridge movies of these procedures prove very helpful. He uses them, essentially, as personal supervisors. He repetitively practices the new techniques while checking himself against the models provided by the films.

Only the close, skilled supervision of his Phase II committee keeps him from becoming so enmeshed in the captivating details of the structural and physiological bases of life as to lose sight of his long-range goals. The most difficult part of this struggle between current enthusiasm and distant objectives in the decision of: how much is enough? The faculty have clearly defined the minimum level of accomplishment that is to be considered acceptable. But, what of the student who is well past this minimum and anxious for more? This is a frequent problem at Metropolitan. Sometimes, much effort is required to help a student gain the difficult professional perspective of balanced personal goals. Further, the faculty believes that, although their curriculum is designed to provide maximum individualization, it is not intended to provide totally free choice. Inherent in the organization of a professional education is the need to clearly specify all areas in which competence is required, if the professional degree and the consequent privileges of licensure are to be awarded. For some students, not all areas of required study coincide with the pattern of their own interests. Most of the time, however, the teachers have no difficulty in assisting the students to see how their inherent interests can find expression in a way that is consistent with the necessary goals of the program.

Before he knows it, Smith's first 18 months of medical school have flown by. Throughout this time the work with Dr. Martin has proceeded rather well. Smith is pleased to look back and realize how much he has begun to understand about many things, ranging from acid-base balance to the psychodynamics of confinement, in the process of participating in the group's research on long-term underwater living.

Phase III of medical school carries Smith through increasing levels of responsibility for patients. The earliest stages are a variey of *simulated* experiences. Much of his basic skill in physical examination is learned on classmates. His first exposure to abnormal physical findings are on both carefully prepared *plastic* models and specially trained *human* models. The non-human models take many shapes. The models of the eye and chest, for example, have in common the versatility of providing the findings of a wide variety of simulated disease states; but they differ in that the eye findings are created by projected images, and the heart and lung findings are synthetically generated electronic sounds which are fed by special amplifiers and dampers to various parts of the artificial chest wall. As Smith looks through his ophthalmoscope into the effectively re-created retina, or listens through his stethoscope, he can operate controls that mimic specific diseases, providing him with experience in identifying particular types of disease findings. By pressing the "random selection" button he is faced with unknowns which test his observational and diagnostic competence.

Several of Smith's Phase III committee members work closely with him in these initial stages. Some of the skills he is learning require their close supervision, either individually or in small student groups. Further practice of these techniques, however, can be checked against the cartridge-film demonstrations and observations by fellow students. Some portions of the physical exam, such as the neurological, are more successfully simulated by human models than by artificial devices. They, too, can provide opportunities for repetitive practice as well as feedback on student success.

By this time, Smith has a fairly good idea of the basics of medical history-taking. But this has come from observation, not performance, and he soon discovers how much more difficult this procedure is than it looks. Of one thing he is already convinced: hardly any aspect of medicine is of more fundamental importance. The diagnostic and therapeutic potential of the clinical history has been amply demonstrated. Together with his committee advisor and a small group of other students, he now begins studying and criticizing prepared video-tapes of history-taking interviews. Then, under observation, the students alternate interviewing trained models. With the fundamentals achieved, Smith next interviews selected patients. He makes video-tapes of these initial patient interviews which are critically reviewed with his instructor. Soon he is sufficiently skilled to derive considerable benefit from reviewing some subsequent tapes on his own, supplemented by occasional cross-checks with his instructor.

Phase III can be viewed as comprised of three parts which shade subtly into each other. With increasing skill at clinical data-gathering (IIIa), he moves to the total study of the pathophysiology of selected patients and of the disease processes they represent (IIIb). Before long, he is moving into the study, and eventually the implementation, of therapeutic programs for his patients (IIIc).

Although the faculty have devoted many years to the refinement of the goals of Phase III, the job is far from done. They have successfully defined many of the diagnostic and therapeutic operations which they feel are fundamental, and they have delineated a basic body of required knowledge. There remains, however, that highly amorphous area which has persisted in defying definition—that area which is commonly labeled, "the doctor-patient relationship." The nagging question is: how does one define the minimal level of acceptable behavior in this area?

The faculty have agreed that every effort must be extended to assure that all students in the school behave in a responsible, ethical manner, that their attitudes toward patients are characterized by kindness and alertness to anxiety and sensitivities, and that they are committed to considering the comfort and convenience of patients ahead of their own. The faculty recognize that criteria for judging student performance in this area are elusive, and that they must avoid the trap of relying exclusively on other, more easily measured aspects of student achievement, such as knowledge of disease. Their approach is to undertake frequent, direct observations of student-patient contacts. By accumulating multiple readings on those student characteristics subsumed by the term, "doctor-patient relationship," they can be reasonably confident of the validity of their judgments.

In the end, the faculty find they can feel fairly certain that Robert Smith and his fellow graduates will serve creditably in their new roles as physicians. Most assuring, probably, is the fact that each has now had several years of experience in assuming the major burden of responsibility for the direction and depth of his own learning; and each has proven, under close scrutiny, to be more than equal to the task. It seems reasonable to assume that they will sustain these attitudes and skills throughout their professional lives.

With graduation only days away, Smith reflects on the years he has spent at Metropolitan, finding that his undergraduate medical education can be viewed as a conceptual whole. From beginning to end it has been a carefully conceived, developing, interrelated sequence. At the outset he was provided with a clear picture of the task ahead and of the goals and standards he was to achieve at each step along the way. Insofar as was possible he generated a highly individual program in which he proceeded at his own speed, using his own interests as a guide to those specific tasks and research projects through which he was able to gain the understandings and acquire the skills which the faculty had defined as necessary. He found himself eager to administer the frequent tests through which he maintained a running check on his success at learning all he wished to know. He suddenly realized how irrelevant now were the old notions of student grades and class ranking. As he indulged in this reflection he was struck with the amusing thought that this entire course of study could be conceived as a grandly elaborated version of what he had heard was once a novel approach to the organizational and educational features of short learning sequences, which went by the name of "self-instructional techniques in medical education."

Is all this a wild, improbable fiction? Possibly. I would contend, rather, that everything we now know makes this little fantasy both an attainable and desirable prospect. The understanding we now have of the processes of human learning must have implications beyond the design of, say, a programmed text in blood clotting or a self-instructional film on child development. The elementary, secondary and college programs now existing in some places and on the horizon in others will be creating students of a quality we have not heretofore dared imagine. I have tried briefly and roughly to sketch a program that may enable the fulfillment of some of the enormous potential such students will bring.

I propose that we already know enough about the design of total educational programs to develop both the environments and the materials which students of this quality need and deserve. The fact is that many parts of this not-so-implausible future are already lurking in our midst. The time seems to be at hand when we can and should extend ourselves to hasten the arrival of this future.

Part II

The Process of Analyzing Self-Instruction

A major concern of any instructor investigating the possibilities of self-instruction involves the selection and evaluation of materials in terms of their utility for his own students. Deterline proposes a framework for analyzing learning programs as a basis for their selection and instructional use. Mager discusses the currently employed criteria for evaluating self-instructional materials, and proposes an improved approach to making critical judgments concerning the value of a learning program. Richardson discusses the specific problems of evaluating self-instructional units in medical education, and reports the beginnings of a system for behavioral analysis that could lead both to clearer identification of instructional objectives and assessment of their attainment.

Selection of Programs

WILLIAM A. DETERLINE, Ph.D.*

THE QUESTION, "What program should I use?" should not be the first concern of a teacher contemplating the possible applications of instructional technology to an educational problem. Rather, the first question should be, "Why should I consider selecting a program, or any other instructional device or medium or method, in the first place?" The answer has to be that there is some existing instructional requirement for which teaching materials or methods of some sort are appropriate.

Still far removed from the possibility of using a program, we must also take a close look at the instructional environment. For example, how do we know that we have an instructional requirement? Where did it come from? Who told us about it and how long ago? To what specialty does it relate, and to what kinds of task performance should it be related? In some cases, it is not possible to determine where the instructional requirement came from or who stated it. We may find that this course has always been taught *this* way, using *these* methods, and containing *this* content, with little justification other than historical precedent.

How long has it been since someone looked at this educational requirement and its content to see how closely they are related to the *performance* requirements of the specific task? When was the last time we did any kind of behavioral task analysis to determine whether the content is directly related to, and completely covers, the perform-

*President, General Programmed Teaching Corporation, Palo Alto, California.

ance requirements of the task? We cannot possibly decide whether or not to select a lecture, a programmed textbook, an audiovisual device, an evaluation instrument, a simulator, or any other component of instruction until we know the behavioral characteristics of the tasks (diagnosing illness, instituting therapy, etc.) for which the instruction is supposedly designed.

Any existing training course, or any course design for a new instructional requirement, should be based on a thorough analysis of the job performance and the environmental characteristics in which the job is to be performed. Robert Mager,[1] in his book on objectives, told a fable, the moral of which is this: If we do not know where we are going, we may end up somewhere else. I would like to stretch that thought even further: If we do not know where we are going, we may end up somewhere else, and not even know it! We need to specify objectives at least to the extent of identifying: (1) the key questions the student should be able to answer; (2) the problems he should be able to solve, and the nature of the solutions; and (3) the situations which require particular kinds of action, together with a description of what constitutes appropriate action. We cannot intelligently proceed with the selection of any instructional device, method, or medium until this information is available to us. The complexities of medicine will often force us to compromise our behavioral analysis, but the more closely we can define and specify our objectives, the more effectively can we design our instructional approach.

Assuming we know what it is we want to teach, we must still examine our existing instructional environment. To what extent is the present course accomplishing each of its instructional objectives? Seldom, if ever, is an educational sequence so well designed, programmed or otherwise, that every student attains every objective. The course may still be considered effective, however, if a significant number of students attain a significant number of objectives. A prime concern for any investigator examining an existing course is this question: in what areas is the course deficient?

There is still another way in which we must examine the instructional situation with which we are concerned. All instruction is designed to change behavior. How much do we know about the behavior of the students at the time they enter our course of instruction? We frequently find that over the years the entering behavior of the students changes, usually upwards; the students may actually bring with them many of the learnings that our course of instruction is designed to teach. For such students, a good deal of teaching is wasted. We ought to have some form of pre-instructional testing in order to compare final criterion performance with entering behavior, to determine exactly how much of a change in behavior we have produced. This means we need to look not only at the objectives of instruction but also at the educational background and personal characteristics of the students entering the course.

It may appear that an inordinate amount of work is necessary just to select a program. I submit that unless we do this work, we might just as well choose a program by flipping a coin. Until we know most of the things I have mentioned, our judgment will be based more on luck than skill. The kinds of information described above are necessary any time we are planning to revise or institute a course of instruction. Indeed, this applies to adding a new textbook, a new audiovisual component, a new testing instrument, or making any other change. Even if we are not planning changes, we should obtain this information periodically to find out if changes are needed. The examination of a course of instruction should probably take place at least once, and preferably twice, a year.

Let us suppose we have this information before us, and we have determined that the content of the instruction is very closely related to the tasks for which it is preparatory. The next step is to compare the stimulus and response aspects of the task with the requirements of the course of instruction. Let me cite an extreme example to illustrate this point. Suppose you have spent many hours observing skilled skiers on the slopes, trying to define precisely the behavior involved and the probable external and internal stimuli to which specific responses must be related. From this data you then write what we call a behavior blueprint, specifying all of the stimulus and response components of the behaviors that you observed the skiers performing. When a student finished going through a paper and pencil program based on the blueprint, he could probably discuss skiing quite knowledgeably. But would you expect him to be able to put on a pair of skis for the first time and perform in such a way that you could say, "That man is a good skier?" Of course not; no more than we could expect a man to become a skilled physician from reading books about medicine. One cannot learn to ski or to practice medicine sitting at a desk. The course of instruction would simply not be related closely enough to the performance requirements.

There are a variety of instructional objectives to which these considerations apply. Physician performance, for example, includes many kinds of behavior: there are behaviors called cognition or perception; there are behaviors related to stimulus discrimination and response differentiation; others related to verbal behavior; others concerned with manipulation of objects and equipment; and still others involving interpersonal relations. In addition, there is a hierarchy of behaviors which must be taken into account in analyzing any course of instruction. For example, teaching an individual to verbalize how to palpate a liver does not necessarily mean that he can do it adequately. Teaching an individual to *discriminate* positive examples from negative examples may not teach him to *produce* positive or correct examples. Conversely, teaching the actual performance of a task may not develop an ability to verbalize the components of that performance. This is illustrated by the centipede which was asked to describe the procedures by which he kept his many legs from getting in each other's way. As soon as he began to think about it, he found himself completely unable to walk. We have to look at all the components of task performance to ascertain if the instructional characteristics actually reflect the range of behaviors called for in the life situation.

Selecting a program, then, depends on an analysis of our objectives, together with an analysis of existing instruction. These analyses are required whether we are developing a new program or evaluating an existing one. Suppose the existing program fits only part of our objectives. We can use it and supplement it with other types of instruction; or we can design a new program to fit our needs, or develop short sequences to be used in conjunction with the program we have just evaluated. We may, if we are lucky, find a program which exactly matches all of our instructional requirements.

There are still other considerations. Is it possible to use the program? It may, for example, be a visual program. Is appropriate space available for its use? What about the cost of the program and the cost of equipment? Are these relevant considerations? Sometimes they may be. What implementation problems might a self-paced program cause? When students proceed through a program on a self-paced basis they will complete the course at different times. Can we handle the scheduling problems involved? Some instructors use a technique called pre-scheduled self-pacing; the students are given a certain amount of material to complete each day. Within that day's assignment, they can schedule themselves on an individually paced basis. Some programs are designed for group classroom use, and they produce other scheduling problems.

Let me now approach this question in a different way. The varying advantages of self-instruction are important to us in the process of selecting a particular program. Programs can produce a gain in amount of learning, greater course coverage, a savings in time, and an elevation in the mean level of achievement. Programs allow us to lower the grade level, that is, deal with younger or less well prepared students. Programs can eliminate drill and routine by teachers, freeing them for other activities. Programs can reduce the failure rate and increase the amount of independent study time. Well-designed programs can increase motivation and morale, influence attitudes, increase retention, and allow fuller use of the capabilities of brighter students.

In some cases, a program may provide only one of these advantages. It may only save time. Or it may not save any time; it may, in fact, take even longer, but produce a significant increase in the amount of learning. It may only increase retention. It may do nothing except reduce the amount of instructor time. We cannot tell these things by looking at a program. We may get some idea of the possible advantages by looking at the data that come with the program. Generally, the only way to get all the necessary information is to try the program out with a small group of students or trainees. We can then test them on our performance objectives and evaluate most of the factors noted above. Have the trial students achieved the objectives adequately? How well do they compare with students coming out of the existing course? How long did it take them, compared to the existing instruction? By looking at each of these factors it can be determined how much we have lost and how much we have gained. We may find, for example, that the program we are considering takes longer than the existing course of instruction, so that we are sacrificing some efficiency in terms of time. Have the gains in other respects compensated for this? There is no objective formula for deciding this; only the individual instructor can make the decision.

Clearly, the selection of a program can be a complicated process. If the procedures outlined above are followed, the limitations of a program will become apparent. If a program is too long, too ponderous, too poorly written, too unrelated to the objectives, or provides too few gains to be worthwhile, these problems quickly come to light.

To review: in selecting a program, there are several steps. First, inspect the instructional requirement, its content, and its general purpose. Second, analyze the existing course of instruction to see if it is related to the behavioral requirements of the task for which it is preparatory. Third, relate the visible objectives of the program to those same task requirements. Sometimes the criterion examination that accompanies a program will identify the objectives. Sometimes you have to learn what they are by inspection. And, in some cases, you can determine the objectives only by taking the program. Fourth, attempt to determine whether or not the stimulus and response characteristics of the program are related to the task, and whether you can expect transfer of skill learning from program to task. Fifth, if the program appears to pass these tests, I would suggest that you have a small group of students try it. Now evaluate the finished product as well as you can in terms of all possible gains, and balance the pluses against the minuses. At this point, the data will generally speak for themselves, and your decision will be made automatically.

In some ways selecting a program is much more precise than selecting a textbook. To properly select a textbook, or any other component of instruction, the full procedure outlined above should be followed. Programs, however, are not books; they do not simply present information. They are designed specifically to change behavior, and they should be selected on the basis of the change in behavior they produce, compared to the final behaviors which are your instructional goals.

The problems involved in selecting off-the-shelf programs have led many teachers to conclude that suitable programs do not and are not likely to exist. The local requirements, procedural policies, or constraints often make programs produced elsewhere unusable in a specific situation. In some cases, it is possible to use part of a program, supplemented by additional instruction of another sort. Sometimes the difficulties are the result of poor selection of content with only limited determination of the needs of the target group. Programs, as they have been and are still being written, are fairly inflexible, so that the user has little chance of "stretching" a program to fit his specific requirements.

One solution appears to be the establishment of a local inhouse programming capability. A number of medical schools have turned to this means of obtaining programs tailored to their needs, but success and satisfaction with this solution has not been universal. Local programming may temporarily cause more problems than it solves, but it may be the best approach in the long run.

There is another approach to the same problem. This depends on the present sources of programs, publishers, programming companies, and local programming operations. The approach takes us back to our subject of objectives. It might be possible for a clearinghouse such as the one in operation at Rochester to function not only as a disseminator of information *to* other medical schools, but also as a collector of information *from* those same institutions about their precise needs. A source of information of this sort could contribute significantly to the determination of an existing "common core" of needs within or across subject matters and performance task areas. Perhaps this could lead to the design and production of small programmed packages which would be responsive to identified needs, and which might, in turn, eliminate most of the selection problems.

References

1. Mager, R. F. *Preparing Objectives for Programmed Instruction.* San Francisco: Fearon, 1961.

Criteria for Evaluation

ROBERT F. MAGER, Ph.D.*

WHAT I PROPOSE TO DO during this discussion is to consider some of the *measures,* as distinguished from procedures, currently used to evaluate the effectiveness of a self-instructional program, to discuss some of the *measures* used in the diagnosis of program weaknesses, and to make a comment or two on the field-testing of programs. Though discussion of the problems of test construction, or of internal and external program characteristics, or of the theory of evaluation procedures, is relevant, these subjects will not be treated here.

If I am successful, you will be able to answer the following questions at the end of this paper:

1. What are the most common currently used criteria for assessing program effectiveness?

2. What measure of program effectiveness appears to be the best of those now commonly in use?

3. What are three useful measures in the diagnosis of program weaknesses?

4. What are the two concepts of field testing, and which appears to be the most useful?

When we talk about measures used in evaluating a self-instructional program we should be talking about the same measures used in evaluating a lecture, or a textbook, or an instructional film. After all, instruction is a process that is intended to change the behavior of a human organism, and the behavior-changing success of one in-

*Director, Behavioral Research Laboratories, Xerox Corporation, Rochester, New York.

structional technique ought to be assessed by the same criteria as are applied to any other instructional technique. Unfortunately this is not the case. We find that people insist on asking questions of self-instructional techniques they have never thought to ask of the other instructional procedures they use. For example, they ask whether a self-instructional program works, when they have never asked this question of their textbooks. They ask whether a self-instructional program achieves the objectives set out for it, when they have never actually enunciated specific objectives for their own lectures and courses. They ask whether a self-instructional program teaches faster than some other techniques, when they have no idea how rapidly these other techniques teach, or might teach, or should teach. They have the temerity to ask whether a self-instructional program teaches creativity, when they have not the slightest idea how they would measure this attribute, even if it occurred to them to ask this question of the instructional techniques they are currently using.

It is not that it is inappropriate to ask these questions of an instructional program; these are precisely the kinds of questions that must be answered if we are to assess the effectiveness and usefulness of the process. But the *same* questions ought to be asked of *any* instructional technique.

Therefore, let us approach our discussion of criteria for evaluating self-instructional programs with the thought in mind that these criteria are appropriate for evaluating the success of any instruction.

What do we want to know?

In discussing valuation criteria for self-instructional programs, let's begin with the rather simple-minded question, "What is it that we want to know about the program?" Once we decide what we would like to know about a program we can proceed to invent or arrange ways of gathering the necessary information. Let's keep in mind that we need to take as many measurements as there are attributes to be measured.

If behavior-changing is the primary purpose of a program, then the *main* criterion we should be interested in is one that tells us something about just how much behavior the program has changed. This implies a *measure of change* from some initial behavior state to some terminal behavior state. Since a measure of change can be made only by making at least two observations at two different points in time, a suitable criterion is one that reflects some sort of difference between "before the program" behavior and "after the program" behavior.

One such measure is the gain score. The simple gain score reflects the difference between a pretest and a post-test score in terms of a percentage (figure 1). For example, if a post-test score were 90 percent and a pretest score 20 percent, the simple gain score would be 90 minus 20 or 70 percent.

FIGURE 1

Gain Score = Post-Test - Pretest

The numbers from which the simple gain is usually derived are the total count of correct answers on before-and-after criterion examinations designed to assess the degree to which the students' behavior approximates the ideal final behavior called for in the specification of terminal objectives. This measure of change might reflect behavior in relation to subject matter, motor skills, attitudes, or motivation. The meaningfulness of a simple gain score is, of course, a function of the degree to which the test items reflect the desired terminal behaviors, and the degree to which the items themselves are examples of good item-writing practice. The point, however, is that the gain score is a comparison of a student's pre-instruction behavior with his post-instruction behavior; it is a comparison of a student with himself. It is not a measure of how much better a student managed to perform than his chance neighbor, nor is it a measure of where a student may happen to fall with respect to some sort of group performance curve. The gain score is a measure of behavior change within a single student and is not influenced by the performance of contemporaries who may actually be noticeably superior, or inferior, to that student.

While this simple difference score is more useful than a single post-test score, it does not properly take into account the fact that a gain from zero to 10 percent is not the same as a gain from 90 to 100 percent. A more sensitive measure of behavior change is needed, and one such measure is found in the modified gain score which places the actual behavior change obtained in a setting of the total possible behavior change (figure 2). That is, it tells us how much of the *possible* improvement was actually realized, thereby compensating to some extent for the problem of unequal difficulty along the gain

FIGURE 2

$$\text{Modified Gain Score} = \frac{\text{Post-Test} - \text{Pretest}}{\text{Maximum Score} - \text{Pretest}}$$

continuum. For example, if as a result of working through a program one student improved from 10 percent to 20 percent, and another student improved from 80 percent to 90 percent, the simple gain score of both students would be 10 percent (figure 3).

FIGURE   3

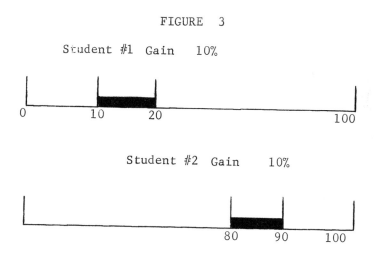

The modified gain score, on the other hand, would show a different picture. Since student #1 traveled only a short distance along the road of possible achievement his modified gain score is much lower than that of student #2, who traveled half the distance from where he was to where we wanted him to go. Substituting values in the formula, we find that student #1 achieved a modified gain score of 11 percent (figure 4).

FIGURE 4

Student #1

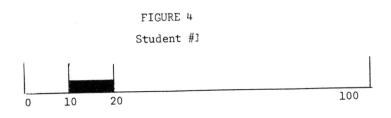

$$\text{Modified Gain} = \frac{20 - 10}{100 - 10} = \frac{10}{90} = 11\%$$

For student #2 the calculation gives a gain score of 50 percent (figure 5). The difference between the scores obtained by these two students reflects the considerably unequal difficulty of achievement for the different levels at which they were working.

FIGURE 5

Student #2

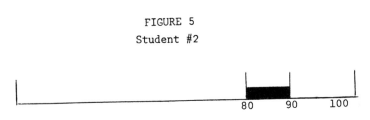

$$\text{Modified Gain} = \frac{90 - 80}{100 - 80} = \frac{10}{20} = 50\%$$

While the simple gain score is one measure of change, the modified gain score is a more sensitive reading and the best that is currently available. It is important to obtain a separate modified gain score for *each* one of the program objectives, using a measure suitable for each.

Assuming we have a measurement that tells us how much behavior a program manages to change, what else would we like to know about the program? Two items devolve from our previous discussion. While a modified gain score tells us something about the effectiveness with which a program manages to change behavior, it does not tell us anything about the nature of the behavior the program is intended to produce, nor does it tell us which behaviors were actually produced. No matter how much behavior is changed, the change is of no value to us unless we are confident that the program is teaching what it is intended to teach, and that what it is *intended* to teach is what we *want* it to teach. We therefore cannot evaluate a self-instructional program until we know the program's objectives, and until we know we have a criterion examination that accurately reflects those desired terminal behaviors (figure 6).

When we *have* the objectives of any program in front of us, that is, when we have a picture of what this unit is intended to do, we can evaluate the program by comparing what it *does* with what is *intended*. In the absence of such objectives we are forced to use such unsatisfactory evaluating techniques as testing each student on the content presented in the program, and comparing one student's progress with that of another. The first procedure is equivalent to taking questions from the end of a textbook; the second is equivalent to grading the students on a curve.

A more appropriate procedure is to define the terminal behaviors desired, construct a performance test that reflects and assesses the existence of these terminal behaviors, administer the test before and after the student works through the program, and then calculate one or more modified gain scores to determine the amount and kind of behavior actually changed. The gain score is not the only useful criterion for assessing the effectiveness of a self-instructional program. When it is intended that a program achieve certain behavior changes within a fixed amount of time, then the amount of time actually required to complete the program must be taken into consideration. When it is intended that certain behaviors be exhibited by the student some time after the completion of instruction, then a measure of retention is needed. In any case, the critical measures appropriate to a given situation are suggested by the program objectives.

One of the evaluation standards currently in vogue is the so-called "80–80" or "90–90" criterion. These numbers imply, for example, that 80 percent of the target population will score at least 80 percent

FIGURE 6

Program Effectiveness Evaluation

Question	Answer Determined By
1. What is the program intended to accomplish?	Behavior Analysis or Terminal Objectives
2. Which of these behaviors actually exist?	Criterion Test
3. How much behavior is changed?	Modified Gain Score

on a criterion examination. These percentages vary according to how well the program developer hopes the students will perform on the terminal examination. Frequently, no pretest is ever given. Such a standard is better than nothing at all, but it must be recognized that this measure is an assessment of how many criterion behaviors are exhibited rather than how many have been *learned*. With the "80–80" approach there is an implication that students could not perform at that level until they had completed the program. The question of whether students *could* have performed at a specified level before instruction, however, is an empirical one open to test, and the answer should be neither assumed nor left unknown. Certainly we would not think much of a programmer who claimed 80 percent of the students going through his sequence could exhibit 80 percent of the criterion behaviors, if we knew that entering students were *already* able to perform at that level. We would be even more distressed if we learned that some students performed *less* well after the program than they did before. The "80–80" standard alone will never reveal for us these types of program weakness.

Similarly, the administration of a final examination in a more traditionally designed course will never reveal whether students are better, or worse off, as a result of completing the course. That is, the results of a final examination can't tell us if students could have performed at the criterion level before the course began. A critic might suggest that instructors who do not give comprehensive pretests are effectively avoiding any possible challenge to their belief that students are better for taking their course. How many instructors do you know who have compared the performance of a class of students who have attended their lectures with the performance of a class of students who have not? I know of experiments of this type in which there was no significant difference in the performance of the group that attended lectures and the group that did not.[2,4,6] While the authors of these experiments conclude that students who did not attend lectures performed just as well as those who did, one could interpret these results even more pointedly by saying that the existence of lectures added nothing significant to the terminal behavior of the students. My reason for mentioning these studies is to underline the fact that an "80–80" or "90–90" type standard may reveal the behavior that exists, but can obscure the manner or the time at which that behavior was acquired.

Program diagnosis

We have been discussing the kinds of information needed to assess whether or not a program teaches what it is intended to teach. Since we are interested not only in how *well* a program works, but also in why it doesn't work, and in why it *doesn't* work *better* than it does, we should consider the accumulation of diagnostic information.

There are several techniques and criteria used to diagnose program difficulties at successive stages in the program development cycle. The diagnostic testing of a program during its construction can be generally classified under the headings: developmental testing and field testing. The difference between them has largely to do with when, and under what conditions, the testing is accomplished (figure 7).

Developmental testing

Developmental testing generally includes any evaluative procedure applied while the program is still under the control of the program producer. During this phase the person or team developing the program is interested in assessing the materials to ensure that they reach the criteria goals, and in detecting the nature and location of critical program weaknesses so that appropriate improvements can be made. It might be useful to list some of the factors (dependent variables) considered in this diagnosis of program weaknesses.

a) **Error rate.** The most frequently used diagnostic criterion is the percentage of errors made by a student while working through a program. Aside from how well a student might perform on a criterion examination, it is generally considered that a program is in need of further revision if the error rate exceeds 5 to 15 percent. Where frequent errors occur on a single item or single sequence of items, the attention of the programmer is focused upon these parts of the program. He looks to see if information is unclear or misleading, or if the frames are so structured as to call for irrelevant responses.

Error rate is an *internal* feature of a program. It may be useful for diagnostic purposes, but it does not represent a measure of the effectiveness with which a program generates desired terminal behavior. It is inappropriate to use error rate as a measure of how well the program achieves the objectives for which it was designed (even though we frequently see it used in just such a manner).

b) Response latency. A more sensitive diagnostic measure is the time that elapses between the presentation of a stimulus frame and the student's response. With this measure it is possible to detect weak or poor frames even when correct responses are made by the student. If a student, for example, should require

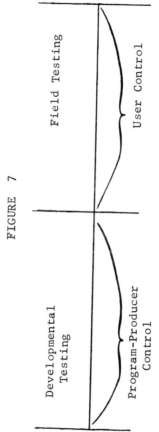

FIGURE 7

considerably more time (perhaps by a factor of 3 or 4) to respond correctly to a frame than he required, on the average, for previous frames, it may be deduced that he was on the verge of an error, that the frame was unnecessarily difficult, or that for some other reason this frame or preceding frames are in need of careful scrutiny. On the other hand further study may show that the frame response simply required more time.

Response latency, like error rate, is a measure of an internal characteristic of the program and is an inappropriate measure of how well a program meets its objectives.

c) **Criterion frames.** Still another measure is the analysis of the criterion frames embedded within the program. These are frames that are normally presented at the end of a teaching sequence and call for the terminal behavior meant to be taught during the sequence. If analysis shows that the desired terminal behavior cannot be elicited even *immediately* after it has been taught, the programmer has a clear indication of program weakness.

d) **Learner attitudes.** While the ultimate purpose of instruction is to modify the behavior of *other* people, it seems reasonable that those engaged in instruction should remain closely in touch with their effect on the student, and that they should demonstrate a willingness to modify their teaching on the basis of what the student has to say. This is generally not the case. Even programmers are beginning to invent ways of avoiding direct contact with, and feedback from, those whose behavior they would change.

Nonetheless, student comments are an important source of diagnostic information. They tell us where the program is too thick or too thin, where the program is written at an inappropriate language level, where the program requires additional examples or practice items; and they tell us whether the program is interesting or boring. In our laboratory, we truly feel that we learn far more during early stages from direct questioning and observation of the student than we do from any of the other measures discussed. It is still true that whenever a programmer experiences difficulty in the development of a sequence, the best approach is to go directly to the student and ask for advice.

Field testing

Developmental testing generally continues until the program is free from reliance on comments and assistance from the programmer, and until it develops in the student the kinds of terminal behaviors desired. In other words, the program is tested until it works under the control of the program developer. Once this point is reached, it is appropriate to determine what needs to be done to make the program work under the control of the intended user. Thus the object of a field test should be not only to find out how well a program *does* work under the control of the intended user, but also, and perhaps primarily, to find out what must be done in order to *make* it work under the control of the intended user.

This last distinction is important. Different field testing procedures are used by those who hold each of these two positions. Those who hold that field testing is merely a validation of the program developed in a laboratory setting, proceed to administer the program to a relatively large number of individuals in the learner's own environment, construct a frequency distribution of criterion test scores, and then publish these data to indicate the general effectiveness level of the program. Those who think of the field test as a procedure for determining what must be done to the laboratory-developed program to make it compatible with, and usable in, the intended environment, proceed more nearly as they did during the early stages of program development. They determine the kind of instructions needed by students and by those who will administer the program, and then draft those instructions until they are as clear as the program itself. They determine the kind of program format or packaging needed to make the program compatible and usable, and test it until it is successful. The intended program user is listened to just as carefully as the student to further increase program compatibility. The point is simply this: it isn't enough to develop and modify a program until it works satisfactorily under the control of the developer; it is also necessary to develop and modify the program until it will work equally well under the control of those for whom it is intended.

Program usability

So far we have discussed some of the criteria used in determining how well a program works, and some of the diagnostic measures useful in attempting to make it work better. In other words, we have discussed ways of proving the pudding and ways of improving the recipe. There is yet a third aspect of program evaluation; there is the consideration of program *suitability*. It is not enough to know that a program works under the control of the program developer, nor is it enough to know that a program will work in the hands of the person for whom it was developed. It is all too possible for a program to be quite effective and very usable, and yet be completely inappropriate or unsuitable in a specific situation. The question of how one determines whether or not a program is suitable in a given situation has been the subject of Dr. Deterline's paper.* I will simply underline our concern with the problem of program selection.

Summary

This paper has been a review of some of the criteria, or measures, currently used in the evaluation of program effectiveness, not of the procedures involved in obtaining these measures. It was pointed out that, since the primary intent of a program is to accomplish behavior change, the primary evaluative technique should be a measure of behavior *change.* To make an appropriate assessment it is necessary to have a clear description of intended behavior change, and performance tests through which the presence of intended behaviors can be detected. These instruments should be administered both "before" and "after," followed by the calculation of as many modified gain scores as necessary to assess the objectives of the instruction. It was suggested that, in addition to measures of program effectiveness, measures of program weakness be used during program development phases. These measures include error rate, response latency, analysis of criterion frames, and learner comments. Finally, it was proposed that if developmental testing means doing what is necessary to cause the program to work under the programmer's control, field testing should mean doing what is necessary to enable the program to work under the user's control.

In a recent discussion with Dr. Matthew Israel on the possible contents of this paper, he suggested an excellent way to summarize the criteria used in the assessment of program effectiveness. He suggested we epitomize the current thinking on program evaluation by saying that those who are behind the times use error rate as the main criterion of effectiveness, those who are with the times use performance test scores, those who are ahead of the times use one or more modified gain scores, and those who are way ahead of the times probably use none of these.

While the evaluation of programs is not a simple process, and while many teachers may choose not to use any of the criteria I have discussed, one thing is clear: as long as we continue to test programs by taking them to the *student* rather than to our colleagues, as long as we measure effectiveness in terms of behavioral outcomes rather than in terms of instructional *process,* we will continue to improve

*Ed. note, see pp. 33-39.

the effectiveness of self-instructional programs. At the same time, we will be learning how to improve the effectiveness of all other instructional procedures.

ACKNOWLEDGEMENTS

To Dr. Bruce Bergum, for his critical review of the manuscript; Dr. Matthew Israel, for his enthusiasm and patience in discussing the content of this paper; and an unnameable programming company, whose ludicrous field testing procedure caused me to devote serious thought to the problem.

References

1. Brooks, L. O. "Student Response: A Guide in Learning Research." Pittsburgh, Pa.: American Institute for Research, September, 1964.

2. Duke, B. C., Jr. "An Analysis of the Learning Effects of Differential Treatment Upon Above and Below Average College Students Enrolled in a Closed Circuit Television Course." Unpublished doctoral dissertation, Pennsylvania State University, 1959.

3. Glaser, Robert. "Instructional Technology and the Measurement of Learning Outcomes." *American Psychologist*. 17:519-521 (August) 1963.

4. Mager, R. F. "On the Sequencing of Instructional Content." *Psychological Reports*. 9:405-413 (September) 1961.

5. Markle, S. M. "Empirical Testing of Programs: Dimensions, Problems, and Issues." NSSE Yearbook (Prepublication draft) March, 1965.

6. Milton, O. Two-Year Follow-up: Objective Data After Learning Without Class Attendance. *Psychological Reports*. 11:833-836 (November) 1962.

Applications to Medical Education

FRED MacD. RICHARDSON, M.D.*

THE ENTIRE EDUCATIONAL PROCESS is inherently self-instructional. This is true despite a great deal of external direction of the student and despite a variety of technical aids supplied to assist him in the process. Although the teacher exerts considerable control through his selection and emphasis of particular content, the student, ultimately, must come to grips with the material according to his own interests, talents, speed, and approach. Student performance on examinations, therefore, reflects some mixture of teacher effects and student capacities. When the teaching and examinations are devised by the same person, there is a risk of restricting the opportunities for students to display accomplishments and limitations which fall outside the perspective of the instructor. This possibility of teacher bias affecting test results was discussed in Green's article, "The Experimental Use of a Programmed Text in a Medical School Course."[1]

In addition, he commented on the use of independently (externally) constructed examinations as they relate to program evaluation, suggesting that "such tests are normally a part of the publisher's field-testing procedures." I would like to emphasize a shortcoming in the approach used, to date, by most publishers. Those tests which have generally been applied to the evaluation of programmed texts have employed items based almost exclusively on the information found in those texts.

*Coordinator of Professional Affairs, The Pennsylvania Hospital, Philadelphia. The Continuation Education Program of the Pennsylvania Hospital receives general support from grants by The John A. Hartford Foundation, Inc., New York.
A portion of this work was accomplished under the terms of Contract #PH 108-64-82 with the Bureau of State Services, Public Health Service, Department of Health, Education and Welfare.

TABLE 1

	Item N	Mean Before	Mean After	Difference
Total Test	181	110.51	114.74	4.23
Objective-Related	104	63.01	67.76	4.75
Non-Related	77	46.70	46.53	-0.17
Programmed Text-Related	27	20.27	21.25	0.98

Student N = 31

When a program is meant to teach a large segment of the core knowledge of a field, the evaluation of its teaching potential must include more. The process falls logically into two phases. The first, validation of the text itself, provides qualitative information on whether or not the text under consideration is effective. This measure must indeed be closely related to the stated objectives of the text, should probably use the language of the text, and might even be considered to consist largely of the set of terminal frames.

The second phase of instructional evaluation must be broadened to measure the relationship between that learning resulting from the use of the text and the total body of available knowledge pertaining to the subject of the text. This quantitative measure can be accomplished only by the use of independently constructed examinations.

Examinations of this type are not often readily available. We in medicine are fortunate in being able to draw upon the item pool of the National Board of Medical Examiners, which can provide a valuable source for the construction of external examinations. Not only are their tests based on sampling over an entire field, but the manner of their construction reflects, to some degree, a national consensus on the body of knowledge appropriate to the level of medical learning being tested. At the First Rochester Conference, Wilds and Zachert reported their use of just such an examination, specially constructed by the National Board, for evaluating the effects of their programmed text on pelvic tumors.[2]

We also have now had experience with "before" and "after" external examinations. These were administered as measures of the effects of a series of postgraduate didactic reviews of obstetrics for general practitioners. "Before" testing of each group of general practitioner students was accomplished with standard Part II National Board Examinations in Obstetrics and Gynecology. For "after" testing, a special examination was constructed by the National Board to match their standard examination both in item number and difficulty. For different student groups, at different times, we used other pairs of examinations, all of which were equilibrated against the original matched pair. Student scores attained on each of the entire series of "before" examinations were found to be so similar that it was possible to study these scores as if they had been derived from a single group experience.[3]

This student group ($n = 56$) attained a mean score on the after examination which was 4.23 points higher than they had on the before examination. This difference was found to be significant at better than the 1 percent level of confidence ($0.01 > p > 0.001$).

In seeking to define more precisely the reasons for this difference, a closer look was taken at the scores made by a smaller sample of students subjected to the matched pair of examinations. A series of teaching objectives was identified from topic outlines submitted by each of the faculty, and the twin National Board examinations were scanned for test items relating to these identified teaching objectives. Item analyses of scores of the 31 students taking these examinations yielded 2 sub-scores; one of these scores came from items related to the teaching objectives, the other from non-related items. The improvement in group total scores (table 1) was accounted for entirely by the difference on objective-related test items.

This technique provided a clear estimation (in terms of National Board examination scores) of the effectiveness of the teaching method. Because of its usefulness, we plan to apply the same examination technique in evaluating the performance of a group which will study a series of programmed texts in obstetrics. This should be an improvement on our current failure to measure the second phase of evaluation.

The *ultimate* measure of instructional effectiveness, however, lies in the identification of change in student behavior attributable to the educational experience. In postgraduate medical education, such behavioral change must be measured in terms of what doctors actually do in the care of patients. Measurement of behavioral change goes a step further than the measurement of cognitive change alone. It examines both intellectual change and its actual application to the doctor-decision process.

A primary requirement for the measurement of change in behavior is a pre-established standard. A major criticism of Peterson's,[4] Clute's,[5] and Trussell's[6] studies of clinical practice was the relative subjectivity of their methods. The establishment of a set of performance standards (or action criteria) before an attempt to measure behavioral change in a study group would significantly increase the objectivity and usefulness of these measures. The definition of such criterion behaviors in the patient-care areas of postgraduate teaching is a prerequisite for the measurement of differences between pre- and post-course physician performance.

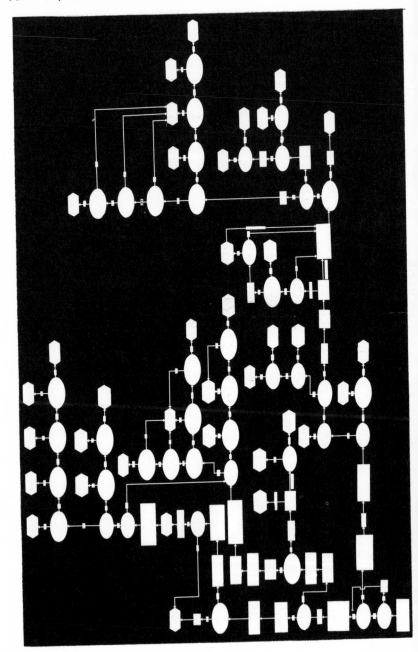

We have developed certain definitions of criterion performance through the analysis of the patient-care procedures of specialists. Behavioral analysis, once obtained, can be seen as a system of information-processing. The patterns of the specialists represent a standard against which the office and hospital records of a study group engaged in the care of similar patients may be compared. If this comparison of the study group's performance is made both before and after the educational experience, the effect of the instruction can be directly estimated.

The criterion performance for the care of patients with third trimester vaginal bleeding was established by the obstetrical staff of the Pennsylvania Hospital. It is summarized as a flow chart in figure 1. Physician procedure in the care of a single patient must be selective, and the care of no one patient involves all of the alternatives here represented. The flow chart, however, provides for all the contingencies found over a wide range of patients, and characterizes the standard performance of the specialist at each step.

As an example of the functioning of the flow chart (figure 2), we can follow the management of 13 patients with a discharge diagnosis of partial placenta previa. All experienced painless vaginal bleeding during the third trimester of their pregnancy. Three of the patients were primiparas and 10 were multiparas. One of the primiparas showed a breech presentation on placentogram. She underwent immediate cesarean section. The other 2 primiparas also had cesarean section, one because her cervix was not sufficiently effaced and dilated to permit quick delivery and the other because fetal vertex remained high in the pelvis despite adequate dilation of the cervix. Nine of the 10 multiparous patients required cesarean section. The remaining patient had a vertex presentation with uneffaced and almost completely dilated cervix and the fetal vertex in mid-pelvis. Amniotomy was performed, forceps applied, rotation completed, and the baby delivered. A complication resulting from this maneuver was a lacerated cervix caused by the forceps. The bleeding from the partial placenta previa, however, was contained, and the placenta delivered with no further hemorrhage and no further loss of circulation to the baby.

There was one discrepancy between the theoretical flow-chart of criterion performance and the actual performance of the criterion staff. They, on observation, proved to be much more inclined to per-

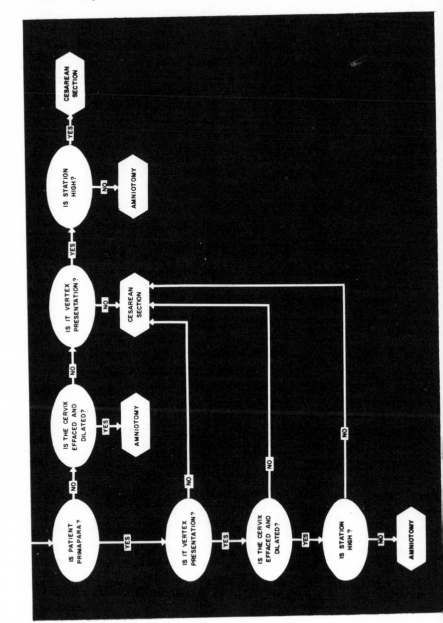

form manual vaginal examinations under sterile conditions than they were to use the speculum examination described on the flow chart. This difference remains to be explained. In any event, only through the establishment of the behavioral analysis could such deviations or discrepancies be identified, let alone investigated.

Meaningful evaluation of the teaching of patient-care procedures requires the behavioral study of what physicians actually do with patients. Objectivity requires the prior establishment of action standards. While initial attempts at behavioral definition will likely omit some of the nuances of physician action, any steps that are taken in the direction of clearer definition of the clinical process will considerably enhance our capacity to provide effective instruction and to assess its outcomes.

References

1. Green, E. J., Weiss, R. J., and Nice, P. O. "The Experimental Use of a Programmed Text in a Medical School Course." *J. Med. Educ.* 37:767-775 (August) 1962.

2. Zachert, V., and Wilds, P. L. "Research Results of a Year's Use of an Adjunctive Linear Program" in Lysaught, J. P. (ed.) *Programmed Instruction in Medical Education.* Rochester, N. Y.: The University of Rochester, 1965.

3. Richardson, F. MacD. "Examinations as Devices for Evaluation." *J. Med. Educ.* 40:972-977 (October) 1965.

4. Peterson, O. L., Andrews, L. P., Spain, R. S., and Greenberg, B. G. "An Analytical Study of North Carolina General Practice." *J. Med. Educ.* 31: Part 2 (December) 1956.

5. Clute, K. F., *The General Practitioner: A Study of Medical Education and Practice in Ontario and Nova Scotia.* Toronto, Canada: University of Toronto Press, 1963.

6. Trussell, R. E. *et al.* "The Quantity, Quality and Costs of Medical and Hospital Care Secured by a Sample of Teamster Families in the New York Area." New York: Columbia University Press, 1959.

EDITORIAL DATAGRAM:

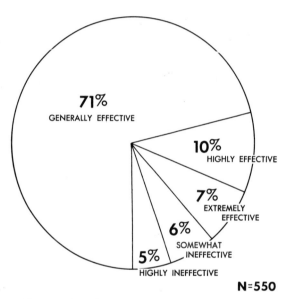

Figure 4. Cumulative results of programmer training at the University of Rochester.

Summary Results of the Training of Teachers As Programmers. For a discussion see the *Bulletin of the Clearinghouse on Self-Instructional Materials for Health Care Facilities,* Vol. 2, No. 1, February, 1967.

Part III

Research on
Self-Instructional Materials

With the first wave of interest in self-instructional techniques for medical education, it was predictable that there would be glowing promises and searing predictions of their impact on curriculum and teaching. In place of the optimistic and pessimistic extremes, we are beginning to accumulate a healthy body of research findings that attest to the strengths and shortcomings of the method—at the level of knowledge rather than conjecture. In this section, Reinecke presents a concise report on a study of the effectiveness of programmed teaching against an absolute criterion of performance. Moser and her associates discuss a classical comparative approach to determining effectiveness, while Wilds and Zachert report a continuing longitudinal study. Some measure of the generality of the results obtained is provided by the studies of Daufi and Fernandez-Cruz in Spain, and of Anderson and his colleagues in England. In sum the papers present a careful and increasingly important documentation of the applications of self-instruction.

Programming in Ophthalmology[1]

ROBERT D. REINECKE, M.D.[*]

GRADUATE MEDICAL education provides a fertile field for self-instructional courses. The students are well-motivated, mature, and highly intelligent. Ophthalmologic training is especially suitable since a large segment of one year is characteristically devoted to didactic study, free of clinical duties. The vocabulary and methodology of ophthalmology are so new and broad as to require extensive didactic courses for the ophthalmologic resident to obtain a firm background prior to his clinical residency. This paper documents the author's experience in developing and testing a self-instructional unit in ophthalmology for residents.

Refraction was chosen as the first subject to program since the instructional goal is clear, and achievement is readily measured. Because our students had no prior ability to execute the skill of refraction, we planned to write a self-instructional course which would enable the students to learn the necessary facts, theories, and rudimentary skills required to perform a basic refraction.

The students

The course was designed for doctors of medicine beginning their specialty preparation in ophthalmology. The students each had a

1. This work was supported in part by U. S. Public Health General Research Support Grant No. RC—1167 from the General Research Support Branch, Division of Research Facilities and Resources, National Institute of Health, U. S. Public Health Service.

*Howe Laboratory of Ophthalmology, Harvard University Medical School and Massachusetts Eye and Ear Infirmary, Boston.

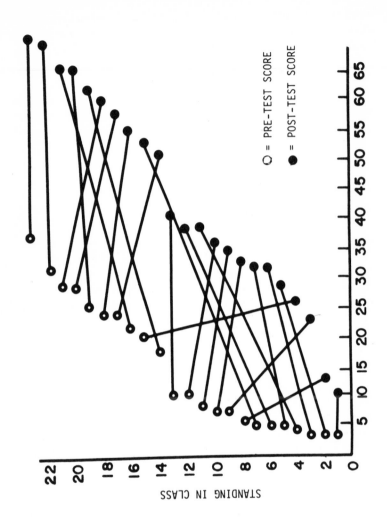

baccalaureate degree, doctorate of medicine, one year's internship, and from zero to three years' specialty training. Within this range of differential training, the program was found to be uniformly effective. The time required for completion of the program varied inversely with the student's prior experience in refraction. Our consideration of the students affected the course design: (1) the material had to be presented with the largest possible steps to prevent boredom; (2) the students were highly motivated and scrupulous in attention to detail, which necessitated that the authors be equally scrupulous in the writing of the program; and (3) the students all were preparing to exercise refraction on patients, so the importance of the subject was obvious to them.

The primary subjects were two successive classes of doctors who were taking a preresidency training course at Harvard. In addition, ancillary medical personnel took the course, but their experience is not reported here.

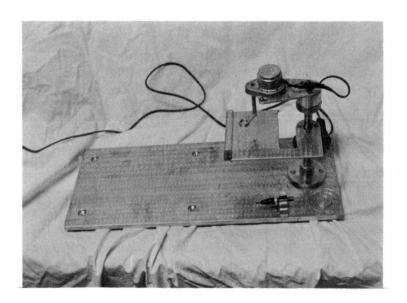

Testing the course

The first class was pretested and subdivided into two comparable groups. One half took the programmed course plus the usual didactic lectures; the other half took only the regular didactic course. Each student was pre- and post-tested on didactic facts as well as on the practical test of refracting a patient (simulated by the author). The students who used the programmed course performed only slightly better on the didactic level, at the p = .15 level of confidence. The practical examination, however, fulfilled all dreams of the author;

only the students who had taken the programmed course were able to do a rudimentary refraction.

The entire second class was given the programmed course before they had any didactic lectures on refraction or its related fields such as optics. Again, the students on completion of the program were able to do a rudimentary refraction. Improvement was also noticeable in these students' participation in the ensuing didactic teaching.

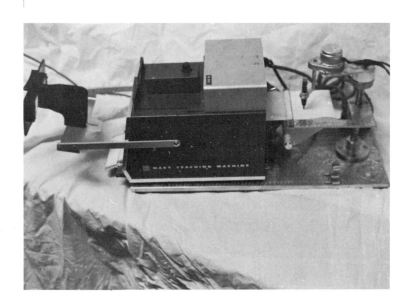

Course content

Basic skills in using equipment were taught, together with that factual and theoretical content important in allowing the student to develop background judgment necessary for the selection of several alternatives in the final prescription. This theoretical content also helped maintain interest in the development of skills. Stereophotos were used extensively whenever the material presented involved three-dimensionality to an important degree. Photos and line drawings were also used liberally.

Special problems were encountered in several areas. Retinoscopy, the objective optical measurement of an eye, utilizes a relatively simple instrument. One difficult feature of retinoscopy, however, lies in interpreting the motion of a reflex in the patient's pupil. Photos of this reflex, together with appropriate drawings, gave the student a sufficiently sound concept of the task to enable him to do a rudimentary retinoscopy with remarkable accuracy on his first attempt.

LATENCY

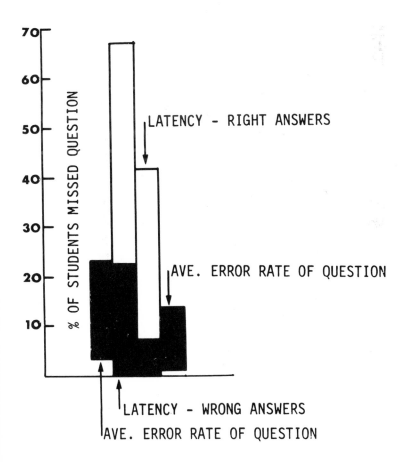

The topography of lenses posed a special problem both in teaching the types of lens surfaces and how to measure them. In the test runs, we used actual lenses, which were satisfactory but expensive. The publication of a text required a choice between mass-producing lenses and using substitutes. We selected the latter. The publisher was successful in arranging for the manufacture of a plastic lens plate which was the anterior and posterior surfaces of lenses molded on one side. The student may use his own lens gauge on these surfaces. In the event that he does not have a gauge, there is an alternate branch which utilizes stereophotos of the lens gauge in use. A small stereo viewer is provided with each published text; the stereo photographs demonstrate the gauge and lens surfaces quite well and dramatically illustrate the topography of the lenses.

The optical properties of the lenses are illustrated with many drawings, but the actual handling of lenses is necessary to establish a working familiarity with them. We assume that every refractionist, or potential refractionist, will have the equipment necessary to do a refraction. Such equipment includes trial lenses. The student is required to use these trial lenses to demonstrate optical properties and to learn the skill of measuring lenses. Teaching a skill to a group of students such as ours requires more than a simple presentation of the act; it requires an explanation of the principle involved. We explain all acts taught, even if they are as simple as measuring the interpupillary distance, using right or left trial lenses, or choosing the hand to hold an instrument. If the principle involved is not overtly taught, we find that the student becomes preoccupied with discovering the omitted reason and does poorly on the following several frames.

Subtle points of simple tasks are included as often as possible. When the measurement and recording of visual acuity was taught, an explanation was presented about the way a patient who has a hemianopsia (blindness of half of the visual field) responds to each line. The student grasped eagerly at the resultant prospect of diagnosing a brain lesion with a test so simple as visual acuity.

Course presentation

The course was a linear program presented on the Mast Teaching Machine. All frames were assigned keysort cards. Each incorrect answer was entered on the card. The students who missed the frame were also noted. A running account was thus kept for each frame, including all incorrect responses, the percentage of students missing each frame, and the identity of the students missing each frame. These cards were used as a basic guide in analysis and revision.

The improvement (post-test over pretest scores) was appreciable in most students. Two exceptions were noted. These two students had prior experience in refraction but were poorly trained. They rebelled against the course, attempting to respond to each question

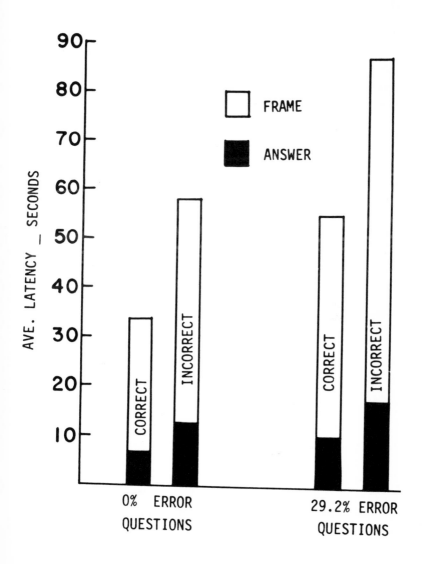

without studying the accompanying frame. Their error rate was extremely high; their improvement was small (see chart 1). Later in the year these two students asked to be allowed to repeat the course. Their answer tape on the second trial was consistent with the first tapes of other tested students, and their final achievement in the clinic was commensurate with their improved performance on the program.

Latency measurements

To measure the latency of student response, we constructed a recorder consisting of a pen which inscribed a circle on the answer tape (figure 1). The Mast Teaching Machine can be placed, without alteration, in the device (figure 2). The answer strip advances each time the student moves to a new frame and each time he uncovers the correct response on the frame, and the resultant tracing of circles permits a close approximation of the time spent on each item.

An analysis of approximately 4,000 frames for latency in respect to: (a) time before the student asked for the correct response, and (b) time spent studying the correct response, showing the following:

Those frames which had an exceedingly low error rate were studied first. The latency of these frames revealed that the longer the time spent on the frame, the greater was the probability of an incorrect response. Similarly, the student spent a longer time studying his incorrect responses.

The incorrect response seemed to act as a remarkably effective means of teaching. One incorrect response often seemed to insure the erring student against making that same mistake again. While I would not advise "programming in" errors or traps, I see no cause to suspect that an occasional error will be a detriment to the student; our observations suggest the reverse.

Those frames which had a high error rate (almost 30 percent) were also analyzed. The same trend was noted except that the students spent even more time on the correct responses than they had on the easy frames, and still greater time on the incorrect frames (chart 2).

The average latency for incorrect responses was almost twice that for the correct responses. The prior cumulative error rate for incorrect responses was approximately twice that of the right responses (see chart 3).

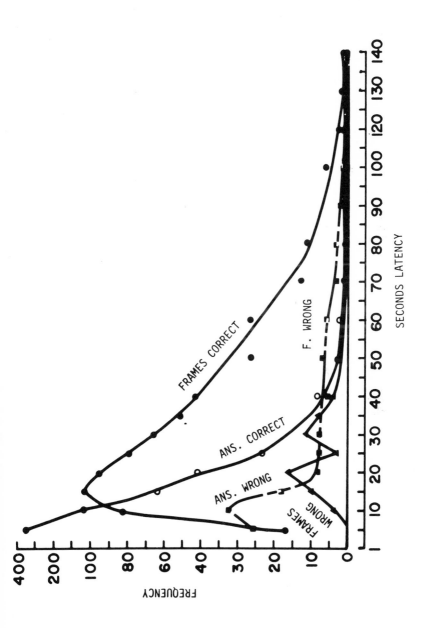

Conclusions

The following conclusions seem warranted by our findings: self-instructional programs seem particularly adaptable to postgradute teaching in opthalmology; skills can be taught readily in areas where the usual didactic work has failed; teaching aids improvised by the programmer and publisher increase the student interest; latency of response is a helpful guide to the need for revision; a long latency period indicates the need for revision and usually parallels a high error rate.

References

1. Reinecke, R. D., Herm, R. S. *Refraction, a Programmed Text.* New York: Appleton-Century-Croft, 1965.

EDITORIAL DATAGRAM:

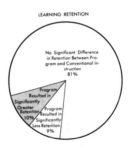

Figure 5. Comparison of Programmed and Conventional Instruction on Retention Measures Only.

Summary Results of Cumulative Studies on Retention in Programmed Instruction. For a discussion see the *Bulletin of the Clearinghouse on Self-Instructional Materials for Health Care Facilities,* Vol. 1, No. 2, July, 1966.

A Comparison of Linear Programs and Lecture Methods in Radiology

PHYLLIS JACKSON MOSER, B.A., R.T.*

CHARLES M. NICE, JR., M.D., Ph.D.**

PHILLIP H. MEYERS, M.D.***

GEORGE R. MECKSTROTH, Ph.D.****

THE ADVANTAGES of programmed education and the ready adaptability of radiology to this format, plus our need for specialized materials for the instruction of students and residents, led the authors to venture into program writing. We identified three areas for which linear programmed texts were then developed: the diagnosis of cardiovascular diseases by x-ray; the diagnosis of lung diseases by x-ray; and radiation protection in a diagnostic x-ray facility. This report describes the development and evaluation of these programs.

Because empiric evidence is the best guarantee of effectiveness, all three programs were subjected to developmental testing. Each program as it reads today is the result of hundreds of hours of writing and of cumulative revision extending over a year and a half. None of the self-instructional texts are intended as reference books; they are courses of study in themselves.

*Research Coordinator
**Professor and Department Chairman
***Associate Professor
****Assistant Professor

All of the Department of Radiology, Tulane University School of Medicine, New Orleans, Louisiana.

Traditionally, Tulane Medical School divides each class of students into small groups, or "blocks," to facilitate teaching and the rotation of students through the various services of the teaching hospital. In their third year, each block of students is assigned to the Radiology Department for a period of regular instruction. Over a period of a year and a half, we used these students to test the programs and determine their teaching effectiveness. From time to time, other groups and individuals used the programs, but the data treated in this paper were obtained solely from the third year students. Since the Tulane medical student may be generally considered to be an average medical student, the results of this extensive period of evaluation have given us a good picture of the effectiveness of our programmed materials.

"Radiation protection in a diagnostic x-ray facility"*

The first program to be completed and tested in the Department of Radiology, "Radiation Protection in a Diagnostic X-Ray Facility,"[1] was designed primarily for the radiologist; but it was written in such a way that medical students and radiologic technologists could also be introduced to the topics of maximum permissible dose, workloads, use factor, occupancy factor, examples of primary barrier computations, and specific instructions for the safety of the operator and the security of the x-ray unit.

A class of 36 junior medical students already scheduled for a lecture on radiation protection were selected as the sample. These students were nearing completion of their course in diagnostic radiology. An explanation of the grouping system was made, and a discussion of the objectives of the experiment followed. All the students were told that they would be given a written test on the material, and that each student's test score would constitute 2 percent of his radiology grade.

Test A (figure 1), a criterion test, was given at the end of the lecture period. Test B, estimated to be approximately equivalent to Test A, was given one week later and was designed to discover any differences in retention of the material. Both Test A and Test B were constructed to measure student grasp of all concepts covered by the basic material.

---

*When the first self-instructional unit written in the department was presented, teaching machines were used with some of the students. Subsequent programs have been developed solely in a programmed text form.

FIGURE 1

SUMMARY OF ACHIEVEMENT TEST SCORES: CONCEPTS OF RADIATION
PROTECTION IN A DIAGNOSTIC X-RAY FACILITY

	GROUP I (LECTURE)	GROUP II (PROGRAM)
	TEST A (end of program)	
MEAN	87.1	86.6
STANDARD DEVIATION	6.24	7.21
RANGE	21.0	27.0
	TEST B (end of first week)	
MEAN	79.1	77.9
STANDARD DEVIATION	9.27	10.39
RANGE	24.0	40.0

Statistical analyses of both criterion and retention test scores revealed that the programmed text was as effective as the method of lecture presentation. (A third group that used the teaching machines earned significantly lower scores when compared with the other two groups.) Analysis of the response errors associated with each frame suggested several points at which minor revisions would probably improve the value of the program as a teaching instrument.

Programmed instruction in cardiovascular roentgenology

The analysis of roentgenograms in cardiovascular disease readily lends itself to the methods of programming. Using actual x-ray films as illustrations, the program we developed consists of a step-by-step breakdown of the circulatory flow, and studies the effects of cardiovascular disease on the pulmonary vasculature and cardiac chambers. This program has been judged by the students themselves to be the most difficult of the three finished programs in radiology, and required an average of 8-10 hours to complete. A self-test is included at the end of the text as an index to the theoretical knowledge gained from this program.

A class of junior medical students was divided into two groups. It was explained that for this experiment one group would hear a traditional lecture presentation of cardiovascular roentgenology, illustrated with 35mm slides and x-ray films, and that the other group would receive identical material, but solely from a programmed text, illustrated with glossy prints of x-ray films. Both groups were informed that they would take the same examination, to be given at the end of the week, and that their score would constitute 25 percent of their radiology grade. We could not, of course, prevent the students in one group from conferring with the students in the other group before the final testing. We did, however, rely on the honor code observed at this institution, together with the expressed willingness of the students to participate in the study comparison, to maintain the protocols and keep the groups separate.

The means for Test A (figure 2), an achievement test, showed an observed difference of 4.3 points, with the program users scoring higher. An analysis of variance[2] provided an F score of 1.38 with one over 39 degrees of freedom. This variance is not statistically significant.

The retention examination (Test B) was given at the end of six weeks. The mean for the group which took the program was 95.2

SUMMARY OF ACHIEVEMENT TEST SCORES: CARDIOVASCULAR ROENTGENOLOGY

	GROUP I (LECTURE)	GROUP II (PROGRAM)
	TEST A (end of first week)	
MEAN	79	83.3
STANDARD DEVIATION	10	10
RANGE	35	30
	TEST B (end of sixth week)	
MEAN	91.1	95.2
STANDARD DEVIATION	5.9	10.5
RANGE	35	20

while the mean for the lecture group was 91.1. An analysis of vari-ance yielded an F score of 1.55 indicating an increased difference between the groups, although still not statistically significant.

Differential diagnosis of lung diseases by x-ray

The program on the differential diagnosis of lung diseases by x-ray was designed primarily for medical students, but we hoped that residents in radiology, and practicing physicians who have some concept of the radiological description and the differential diagnosis of chest lesions, might find the material of some use in review. The data which follow are based on one group of 41 junior medical students who had been assigned to attend a series of radiological lectures on lung diseases. The objectives of the experiment and the division of the students into two subgroups were explained. The students were informed that each group would receive the identical examination at the end of the week and, further, that this examination would include the actual viewing and reading of diagnostic x-ray films displayed on viewboxes.

Test A, the criterion test, was given at the end of the week during which the lectures and the program were presented. The test consisted of 25 questions plus 10 x-ray films which the students were to describe in the radiological terminology they had learned, giving a differential diagnosis of at least three disease processes.

Test B, a practical, was given 6 weeks following completion of the criterion test. It was designed to measure comprehensively the major concepts covered by both methods of presentation, and consisted solely of x-ray films. The students were asked to report their readings of the films in radiological terminology and to give a differential diagnosis of three disease processes for each film. The 10 films used in the test were selected from the 61 which comprise the illustrations for the program. These 10, however, had not been singled out or emphasized more than the other films during the instruction.

To test for possible differences in retention of the material, a different but comparable examination (Test C) was given 12 weeks following the completion of the experiment. This examination consisted of 10 radiographs which were entirely new to the students. A reading of the films in radiological terminology and a differential diagnosis of three disease processes was required.

The results of all three tests (figure 3) were subjected to a simple analysis of variance providing the following F scores: Test A, 2.44;

FIGURE 3

SUMMARY OF ACHIEVEMENT TEST SCORES: DIFFERENTIAL
DIAGNOSIS OF LUNG DISEASE BY X-RAY

	GROUP I (LECTURE)	GROUP II (PROGRAM)
	TEST A (end of first week)	
MEAN	85.6	92.2
STANDARD DEVIATION	5.6	6.03
RANGE	20	22
	TEST B (end of sixth week)	
MEAN	67.1	67.2
STANDARD DEVIATION	21.0	12.04
RANGE	65	48
	TEST C (end of twelfth week)	
MEAN	71	69
STANDARD DEVIATION	8.8	15.2
RANGE	32	48

Test B, 0.187; Test C, 0.513. None of these variances had statistical significance, for which an F score of 4.08 would be required.

Discussion

As they now stand, the three programs we have discussed have been found to be as effective for instructional purposes as the didactic lecture method of presentation. Each program has been revised and rewritten following its administration, in line with the policy of the authors to rewrite any frame having an error rate in excess of ten percent. We do not plan to cease revision now that the programs can be said to be as effective as the lecture. This is not our criterion of excellence. It is our plan to continue revision until the results of the program are demonstrably superior to the results of the lecture method. We feel that further reworking of frame construction could produce significantly higher achievement test scores and improve the educational adequacy of each program.

This presentation would not be complete without some mention of the emotional factors involved in the introduction of programmed material into the curriculum of our department. The reaction of the students ranged from wild enthusiasm to open hostility. Some were resentful at being used as "guinea pigs." Some completely misunderstood the purpose of programmed instruction, feeling that it was designed to replace lecture methods entirely, and might afford the medical faculty an opportunity to withdraw farther from the student-teacher relationship. Others confided their resentment at helping to improve a program which they felt would eventually line the author's pockets with gold.

Our approach of evaluating the programs by comparing the results of one learner group with the results of the other led several students to feel we were trying to "prove" that the program was superior to the regular lecture method. A small band of students reduced the whole issue of programmed instruction to a discussion of the fitness of the radiology faculty to hold their jobs.

Valid criticism can be levelled against some of the methods we were forced to employ in the administration of the programmed texts. Due to lack of space and facilities, students were often crowded around viewboxes on which were displayed the x-rays which accompanied the program frames. The viewboxes lined a well-traveled hallway open to the public, and on a direct line to the library. While some seating was provided in the hallway, the chairs were not at a convenient level for proper viewing of the x-rays. These same facilities had to be employed when we administered the practical tests covering program and lecture material, and the crowded conditions and noisy atmosphere were not conducive to a warm feeling for the Department of Radiology on the part of the students. At times, students passing the department laboratories were heard to express themselves with hisses and boos.

Despite these problems, real or imagined, most of the students appreciated the efforts of the Department of Radiology to improve its teaching methods. In an opinion poll conducted by a student organization, the students reported that programmed instruction *was* a helpful teaching aid. Criticism was restricted to the conditions under which they had to use the programs. Perhaps a better public relations job in selling the advantages of programmed instruction might be in order, to reduce the resentment built up by the somewhat unpleasant field test conditions.

A fourth linear program is now in preparation, with a half-dozen more planned over the next two to three years. Radiology was the first, and remains the only, department at Tulane Medical School to adapt programming to its curriculum. With the recent acquisition of some grant support, we are hopeful of expanding our programming efforts and establishing a programmed education center in the department that would be useful to the entire medical school. At the same time our faculty is critically evaluating our present course offerings with an eye toward a core curriculum in which all topics outside this core would be presented by means of programmed materials.

ACKNOWLEDGEMENT

The senior author wishes to express her gratitude to Dr. S. Thomas Elder, Associate Professor of Psychology, Louisiana State University in New Orleans, for his personal interest and for the significant help he has given.

References

1. Elder, S. T., Meckstroth, G. R., Nice, C. M., Jr., and Meyers, P. H. "Comparison of a Linear Program in Radiation Protection with a Traditional Lecture Presentation." *J. Med. Educ.* 39:1078-1082 (December) 1964.

2. Guilford, J. P. *Fundamental Statistics in Psychology and Education.* New York: McGraw-Hill, 1956.

Effectiveness of Two Programmed Texts in Teaching Gynecologic Oncology to Junior Medical Students*

PRESTON LEA WILDS, M.D.** and
VIRGINIA ZACHERT, Ph.D.***

THE AUTHORS have developed two types of programmed texts to help junior medical students learn the detection, diagnosis, and management of gynecologic neoplastic diseases.

1. An 830-frame linear programmed text covering the "content" of gynecologic oncology in traditional diadactic fashion.

2. A 713-frame text consisting of 35 case presentations of patients with representative types of pelvic neoplasms and related conditions. This text attempts to teach "applications" of gynecologic oncology by the case-study method and contains remedial referrals to the linear text.

First year—"Content" Text

In the academic year 1963-64, the linear text was compared with conventional classroom teaching in a controlled, balanced study at the Medical College of Georgia. Criterion measures of immediate achievement of learning were pre- and post-test examinations of 108 questions each prepared independently for this project by the National Board of Medical Examiners from their pool of questions in gynecologic oncology. The programmed text and the examinations were prepared during a four month period in the summer of

*This work has been supported by a grant from the U. S. Office of Education, Department of Health, Education and Welfare, No. 7-20-0260-219.
**Associate Professor of Obstetrics and Gynecology, Medical College of Georgia.
***Research Psychologist, Department of Obstetrics and Gynecology, Medical College of Georgia.

1963. The writers of the programmed text made no effort to acquire a familiarity with the pool of questions of the National Board of Medical Examiners.

Thus, the programmed text was not written with the special examinations in mind. The objectives of the programmed text had been specified in detail through a series of conferences with members of the Department of Obstetrics and Gynecology, and most of the text was written before any exchange of information took place with the National Board of Medical Examiners.

When the tests were made available, it became evident that questions were asked on the tests which were beyond the scope of our programmed text. We deliberately made no changes in the later revisions of the programmed text to reflect these differences. We emphasize this point because the text was designed to represent our department's teaching policy in the field of gynecologic neoplasms, and was in no sense designed to "teach for the tests."*

The study sample in the academic year 1963-64 consisted of 92 students of the Junior Class. They were divided into four equal groups on the basis of their academic performance in the first two years of medical school. These groups also proved to be comparable in terms of their Medical College Admission Test scores. Each group served a 9-week clerkship in obstetrics and gynecology. They were given one of the National Board's special tests on gynecologic oncology at the beginning of the clerkship and another at the end. Control groups, serving in the first and fourth quarters, were taught by our conventional methods of instruction, which consisted of eight lectures at weekly intervals by one of our senior teachers. Every effort was made to insure that these lectures were of superior quality. They were profusely illustrated with colored slides and other visual aids. At some lectures, mimeographed handouts were provided. All lectures were tape recorded. Attendance at all lectures was required, except when a student had conflicting responsibilities in the operating room or in the delivery room. The average student attended six of the eight lectures.

The experimental groups served their clerkships in the second and third quarters of the academic year. The programmed texts were distributed to them following completion of the pretest. No other formal instruction in gynecologic oncology was provided. The stu-

*Ed. note: see Richardson, pp. 54-61, for discussion of this principle.

TABLE 1

SUMMARY OF RAW SCORES ON SPECIAL NATIONAL BOARD EXAMINATIONS
USED ON PROGRAMMED INSTRUCTION PROJECT AT THE MEDICAL
COLLEGE OF GEORGIA 1963-64

	N	NB Special Examinations Pre-	NB Special Examinations Post-	NB Special Examinations Gain	Study Time (Hours) From All Sources
Control A and A'	45	57.8	85.0	27.2	21.0*
Experimental B and B'	46	56.3	85.9	29.6	21.9
t **		.8	.6		
Significance		NS	NS		

*Does not include 8 hours of scheduled formal teaching.

**Difference mean scores.

dents, however, attended ward rounds, helped care for patients with gynecologic neoplasms, and participated in pathology and tumor conferences just as the control groups did. Both control and experimental groups kept records of how they spent their time studying gynecologic neoplastic disease. They were asked to record their hours attending lectures or classes in gynecologic neoplasms, their hours reading in regular textbooks, reading in other texts or journals, and their hours with the programmed text. They also recorded the number of patients they had been assigned who had gynecologic neoplastic disease. Table 1 represents a summary of our results during the first year of the study. It is apparent that the achievement of the experimental groups is at least comparable to that of the control groups and that they achieved their learning with a saving of nearly all of the lecture time.

Cross-validation—"Content" Text

In the second year of the study, the academic year 1964-65, the experiment at the Medical College of Georgia was subjected to cross-validation studies in five other medical schools. In each of these schools the class was equally divided into control and experimental groups, using methods similar to those employed at the Medical College of Georgia. Experimental groups were given the programmed text. Control groups were taught by their school's conventional methods. The student sample varied among the schools. In one school the students were sophomores. In another the students were seniors. In the remaining three, they were juniors. The methods of conventional teaching ranged from formal lectures, to seminars centered around case presentations, to small group conferences.

The test scores with the gains for the various schools are shown in table 2. The scores show that despite differences in the samples, in the *methods* of teaching used with the control groups, and in the degree of enthusiasm for this project among the faculty of the different schools, the results are quite uniform, clearly favoring the experimental groups. The students at these schools also kept records of how they spent their time studying gynecologic neoplasms. While the data suggest that the programmed text consistently produced more learning than the conventional teaching, the study time differences between control and experimental groups varied so greatly from school to school that conclusions regarding relative efficiency of learning cannot be made.

All experimental group students were asked to complete an attitude questionnaire concerning this programmed text. While they could complete the form anonymously, few students adopted this option. The reaction of almost all students towards this teaching method was favorable, varying from slightly so to all-out enthusiasms. Only a small minority, less than 5 percent in the six medical schools under study, expressed negative reactions. These tended to be students of the highest academic ranking, who found that this programmed text tended to retard rather than improve their already rapid and efficient methods of learning.

Similar questionnaires have not yet been administered to faculty members in the departments of obstetrics and gynecology. The verbal comments, however, from most of the faculty members responsible for this program in the other medical schools, suggested that they have inspected the "content" text and found it unimpressive. It is described as skimpy in its coverage of the subject matter, not always accurate, requiring an unnecessary amount of writing, generally dull, and repetitious. Why such a program should teach better than an experienced, dedicated, live teacher or a far more readable, lively, and authoritative textbook remains to be explained.

In our opinion, the faculty criticisms of our text are reasonably valid. In the first year of our study, however, an earlier version of the text, suffering from considerably more of these very same faults, taught just as effectively. We suspect that the text is effective because it requires the student to develop and use actively the working vocabulary of this discipline. In completing this programmed text, the student learns to express the important facts and principles of gynecologic oncology in his own words. This ability to use the language actively facilitates learning from other sources, such as conferences and conversations with residents and faculty advisors. Familiarity with the language probably also increases efficiency in learning from conventional articles and texts. In our view, the achievement of this text in improving the student's facility with the language of the discipline contributes more to the success of the method than does its presentation of the "content" itself.

Second year—Case Presentation "Applications" Text

In the second year of the project, the academic year 1964-65, we developed programmed materials to teach "applications" of gynecologic oncology by the case study method. We wrote a 713-frame

TABLE 2

SUMMARY OF RAW SCORES ON SPECIAL NATIONAL BOARD EXAMINATIONS
USED ON PROGRAMMED INSTRUCTION PROJECT AT
FIVE MEDICAL SCHOOLS, 1964-65

		N	NB Special Examinations Pre-	Post-	Gain	Study Time (Hours)*
J. of Vermont	Cont.	22	56.8	80.2	23.4	9.8
Medical School	Exp.	23	57.6	85.2	27.6	23.1
	t		.03	2.3		
	Significance		NS	.05		
U. of N.C.	Cont.	11	67.9	84.9	17.0	18.8
Medical School	Exp.	30	61.4	89.3	27.9	25.3
	t**		2.9	2.1		
	Significance		.01	.05		
U. of Nebraska	Cont.	38	61.6	79.8	18.2	11.6
Medical School	Exp.	42	64.6	84.7	20.1	18.1
	t		1.3	2.7		
	Significance		NS	.01		
State U. of	Cont.	45	63.1	88.6	25.5	29.2
Iowa Medical	Exp.	43	61.9	93.3	31.4	29.1
School	t		.1	3.2		
	Significance		NS	.01		
California	Cont.	45	45.5	76.0	30.4	14.5
College of	Exp.	47	47.0	81.0	34.0	22.3
Medicine	t		1.2	3.2		
	Significance		NS	.01		

*Lectures, conferences, demonstrations and wardwork not
included.

*Note that the pretest indicated the control group's mean
was significantly better but post-test indicates significant
gain for experimental groups.

text consisting of 35 case presentations of patients with representative types of pelvic neoplasms and related conditions, each case involving two major phases of patient management.

The first phase is that of gathering information in order to define
the patient's problem or problems. This includes history taking, performance of a general physical examination and various special
examinations, and the selection and interpretation of a wide range
of diagnostic tests and procedures. In case presentations involving

data-gathering, the student is asked to begin with a minimum of information about the patient, often no more than a chief complaint, and collect further information in whatever sequence he thinks is appropriate. The more information he gathers, the more selective he becomes in the acquisition of further information. Also, the more he must call upon and apply his fund of specialized medical knowledge. Ultimately, he must decide when he has collected enough information so that he has defined the problem sufficiently to proceed with the management of the patient.

At this point, he proceeds to the second phase, the formulation of a plan of therapy. After the student has outlined his therapy and has made the important decisions which affect the well-being of his patient, he is told the outcome for his patient. Whenever this outcome is unsatisfactory, he is informed of the nature of his deficiencies and is given remedial advice as to how they may be corrected. Sometimes the remedial instruction is within the case presentation itself; at other times, remedial referrals are made to instructional materials elsewhere, usually in the "content" text.

In the second year of our project, the experimental plan was similar to the first. The students of the junior class were again divided into four control and experimental groups served in the two middle quarters.

The written examinations in gynecologic oncology supplied by the National Board of Medical Examiners were administered to each group as pre- and post-tests in the same manner as during the previous year. These tests were used to measure achievement in the learning of "content." In this second year, no lectures were given in gynecologic oncology. Control students, instead, were given the "content" programmed text, thus receiving the same treatment as the experimental students of the previous year. Experimental groups in 1964-65 received both the "content" text and the "applications" text. Scores on the special examinations (table 3) indicate that "content" was learned as fully and as efficiently without the added "applications" text as with it.

Measuring "application": oral examinations

In both years of this study, the principal measurement of skill in "patient management" or the "application" of specialized knowledge of gynecologic oncology to problems of patient care was a specially devised oral examination administered by a panel of visiting judges

TABLE 3

SUMMARY OF RAW SCORES ON SPECIAL NATIONAL BOARD EXAMINATIONS USED ON PROGRAMMED INSTRUCTION PROJECT AT THE MEDICAL COLLEGE OF GEORGIA 1964-65

| | $\frac{X}{N}$ | NB Special Examinations | | | Study Time (Hours) |
		Pre-	Post-	Gain	
Control A and A'	45	51.6	83.3	31.7	32.6
Experimental B and B'	47	53.7	84.7	31.0	33.6
t **		1.0	.7		
Significance		NS	NS		

** Difference in Mean Scores

and held near the end of the second and fourth quarters. The judges were two visiting professors of obstetrics and gynecology from medical schools in neighboring states. Each student was examined jointly by the two judges in a half-hour interview. Students from the current quarter and those who had served their clerkship during the immediately preceding quarter were presented to the judges in scrambled order. The judges were not informed, nor were they able to determine, the methods of instruction each student had received. The judges were asked to examine each student by presenting hypothetical problem cases to be solved. These cases were to center on problems in the field of gynecologic oncology or related conditions. At the conclusion of each interview, each judge was asked independently to write down immediately: (1) a grade for "content," representing the student's "book knowledge," and (2) a grade for "application," representing the skill with which the student applied such knowledge as he had to the problems of patient care with which he had been presented. After the judges had noted their grades and after the student had left the room, the judges were asked to consult and to reach, by consensus: (3) a final pooled grade, representing their overall judgment of the student's performance in patient management.

The final pooled grade was used as our criterion of "application" in this study. In effect, our oral examiners in a week-long examining session were asked to rate a scrambled group of about 45 control and experimental students on their verbal skills in management of patients with gynecologic neoplasms. It should be apparent that the scoring standards of the examiners would be relative only to the group which they were then examining, and would tend to vary from our examining session to the next as well as from year to year.

It should also be apparent that students who were currently serving their clerkship in obstetrics and gynecology would tend to perform better on the oral examinations than would students who had devoted an intervening two months to the intensive study of general surgery. The experimental plan of the project, with its A, B, B′, and A′ format, permits valid comparisons to be made only at the end of each academic year, when the scores of the two experimental groups and the two control groups can be combined. When this is done, the differences between experimental and control groups in recency of instruction cancel each other out. The design of our project permits only a single comparison to be made each year from the nearly 100 oral examinations conducted.

During the first year of the study, the control group had been taught by conventional lectures and were compared with the experimental groups who had been given only the "content" programmed text. It was our expectation that there would be little difference between these groups in their skill in patient management. The data (table 4) show, however, that in the academic year 1963-64 there was an observable difference between the control and experimental groups in their oral examination scores, although the difference is not statistically significant. This suggests that our "content" text, although not designed to teach "application," may have tended to support learning in this area more effectively than did our conventional methods of classroom instruction.

In the second year of the project, the instructional method which had been found to be the more effective in the first year became our control treatment. Only by this means would we compare the effectiveness of our experimental program in the second year with the one used in the first year. In 1964-65, the control groups received the "content" text with no lectures and the experimental groups received both the "content" text and the "applications" text. The difference in mean scores on oral examinations in the second year of the project favors the experimental groups, but again without statistical significance.

It is not clear from the oral examination results, moreover, whether the slightly improved performance of our experimental groups represented only superior retention of learning or whether these students as a result of their working through the 31 cases, actually developed superior skill in the management of patients with gynecologic neoplasms. Furthermore, it is unclear from the oral examinations what proportional contributions to a given score were made by each of the two factors: skill in patient work-up, and skill in proposing a solution for the patient's problem once it had been defined.

Measuring retention of learning:
National Board Examinations—Part II.

In both years of our project we attempted to evaluate the effectiveness of our programmed texts in improving retention of learning as measured by written examinations. In the spring of 1963 and at the end of each succeeding academic year, we administered the examination in Obstetrics and Gynecology, from Part II of the National

TABLE 4

SUMMARY OF ORAL EXAMINATION "POOLED" GRADES,
MEDICAL COLLEGE OF GEORGIA

	N	1963-64 Mean	SD	1964-65 Mean	SD
Control A and A'	45	2.022	.866	1.933	1.044
Experimental B and B'	46	2.174	.957	2.298	1.021
t*		.8		1.7	
Significance		NS		.10	

*Difference in Mean Score

0 = Unsatisfactory, without reservation

1 = Borderline or questionable knowledge, performance,
    ability, Passing subject to Promotion Board.

2 = Satisfactory knowledge and performance - Average

3 = Better than average

4 = All-round superior student with above average
    preparation, capabilities, performance, interest,
    knowledge, drive, etc.

All oral examinations were conducted by Dr. Michael Newton
University of Mississippi School of Medicine, and Dr. E. J
Dennis, Medical College of South Carolina.

Board of Medical Examiners, to the entire Junior Class. A different
version of this same comprehensive examination was administered
to each class a year later, at the completion of their senior year. This

second test was taken from 12 to 18 months after the clinical clerk-ship in obstetrics and gynecology. In general, the performance of control and experimental groups on these examinations tended to parallel their performance on the written examinations in gyneco-logic oncology specially prepared for this project.

The results for 1964-65 (table 5) indicate that when conventional multiple-choice testing is used, there is little difference in the per-formance of control and experimental groups. There are two pos-sible explanations. The "applications" text may not have significantly altered the students' learning of "content." The similar performance of the two groups may also stem from the fact that the experimental group serving their clerkships in the third quarter of the academic year did not sustain the level of academic performance they had achieved in the first two years of medical school. In *all* written tests in obstetrics and gynecology, this group did relatively poorly.

Final results on retention of learning for the present Junior Class will not be available till after their graduation in June 1966. For all other groups, the National Board of Medical Examiners has supplied us with a categorical analysis of their performance on the final exam-ination in obstetrics and gynecology. The questions were divided into the following categories:

1. Embryology, Anatomy and Physiology of the Female Or-gans of Reproduction.

2. Physiology and Ecology of Woman.

3. Normal Pregnancy: Physiology, Biochemistry, Psychology, Diagnosis, and Management.

4. Physiology and Conduct of Normal Labor and Parturition; the Newborn.

5. The Puerperium; Normal and Abnormal.

6. Complications of Pregnancy.

7. Complications of Labor and Delivery.

8. Disturbances of Function.

9. Anatomic Pelvic Disorders.

10. Infections.

11. Neoplasms.

Category 11 embraces the subject matter of this study. Table 6 presents the scores obtained in each category by all junior students

TABLE 5

RAW SCORE MEANS AND STANDARD DEVIATIONS FOR JUNIOR STUDENTS ON NATIONAL BOARD PART II, AND SPECIAL EXAMINATIONS USED AT THE MEDICAL COLLEGE OF GEORGIA

		NBME Final Grade (May 1964)		Neoplasms Pre-Test		Neoplasms Post-Test	
		Mean	SD	Mean	SD	Mean	SD
1963-64							
A - Control	23	79.1	5.1	52.0	6.9	83.6	7.5
A' - Control	22	83.4	4.6	53.8	7.5	86.5	5.7
B - Experimental	24	79.2	4.2	55.5	7.1	84.7	6.0
B' - Experimental	22	78.9	4.4	57.1	8.2	87.1	7.3
1964-65		(May 1965)					
A - Control	24	78.8	5.4	50.0	9.2	82.2	8.6
A' - Control	21	82.5	3.5	53.4	5.2	84.6	8.8
B - Experimental	24	83.2	4.9	55.4	10.8	86.0	9.6
B' - Experimental	23	80.6	5.2	52.3	11.2	83.3	8.2

TABLE 6

COMPARISON OF MEDICAL COLLEGE OF GEORGIA JUNIOR STUDENTS
WITH NATIONAL BOARD CANDIDATES ON MEAN PERCENTAGES
BY CATEGORY, MAY 1963, MAY 1964, MAY 1965

		MEAN PERCENTAGES				
CATEGORY		Juniors 1963		Juniors 1964		Juniors 1965
(Examination Code)		(KMB)		(LMB)		(0420S)
		NB	MCG	NB	NCG	NB	NCG
1. Embryology, Anatomy and Physiology of the Female Organs of Reproduction		67.3	63.3	72.7	65.5	77.8	66.8
2. Physiology and Ecology of Woman		74.3	65.9	70.0	65.9	75.8	73.9
3. Normal Pregnancy: Physiology, Biochemistry, Psychology, Diagnosis, Management		65.3	62.0	63.1	54.2	77.0	66.7
4. Physiology and Conduct of Normal Labor and Parturition; the Newborn		64.9	63.8	65.0	57.4	71.0	63.0
5. The Puerperium; Normal and Abnormal		66.2	58.7	77.1	64.0	76.0	48.0
6. Complications of Pregnancy		71.9	67.2	69.7	64.8	66.7	57.1
7. Complications of Labor and Delivery		58.3	56.6	68.8	57.9	75.9	69.0
8. Disturbances of Function		63.2	60.4	84.7	76.4	75.3	66.8
9. Anatomic Pelvic Disorders		65.4	60.6	50.0	42.6	83.6	80.0
10. Infections		78.5	71.9	68.9	56.8	52.6	44.3
11. Neoplasms		71.9	62.8	66.2	69.9	67.9	73.7

who took the test during the past three years. In May 1963, before our current project was announced, the test was administered to the Junior Class at the end of the year. As expected, these juniors were below the national average in every category, this average having been derived from the performance of seniors who were taking the examination as candidates for licensure. In May 1964, the examination was administered to the next Junior Class. An exception now appears. In contrast to their scores on all other categories, on "Neoplasms" our juniors were significantly above the national average. The current Junior Class was administered another National Board Examination in May of 1965. Again, only in the category of neoplasms are our students clearly superior to the national average.

Retention after one year

Table 7 shows the categorical analysis for the class of 1965, which took the Examination in Obstetrics and Gynecology, Part II, of the National Board of Medical Examiners, both as juniors and seniors. It is apparent that after the lapse of a year, any differential effects of our teaching in 1963-64 are no longer detected.

Measuring "application" by patient-management examination

To explore further any differences between teaching of patient management by a linear text alone and by teaching with a supplemental text of case presentations, we devoted a set of 9 patient-management examinations. These were in addition to our program of special oral examinations. In constructing our tests, we borrowed ideas and techniques from many sources, including McGuire,[1] Hubbard,[2] and Rimoldi,[3] and developed a special format which gives the student random access to large amounts of information. In each of our patient-management tests, the student is given an opportunity to take a history, do a physical examination, and order diagnostic studies and procedures in whatever sequence he chooses. In most cases, he may collect data on more than a hundred different items. In each test he is asked to define the patient's problem in detail, specifying the patient's primary diagnosis, the extent of her disease, and her various complicating and subsidiary diagnoses. He is also asked to select from as many as fifty possibilities a plan or plans of treatment appropriate to the patient's problems, as he has defined them.

TABLE 7

NATIONAL BOARD MEAN PERCENTAGES BY CATEGORY, COMPARING
MEDICAL COLLEGE OF GEORGIA STUDENTS AT END OF
JUNIOR AND SENIOR YEARS

Category	NB (LMB)	MAY 1964 Junior Year		NB (70420S)	MAY 1965 Senior Year	
		Control	Experimental		Control	Experimental
1	72.7	64.5	66.5	77.8	53.8	63.6
2	70.0	67.1	64.7	75.8	61.1	63.2
3	63.1	54.7	53.7	77.0	61.6	61.4
4	65.0	59.8	55.1	71.0	63.5	61.7
5	77.1	64.9	63.1	76.0	27.0	44.0
6	69.7	67.7	62.1	66.7	54.1	52.4
7	68.8	62.0	53.9	75.9	63.4	61.5
8	84.7	75.5	77.3	75.3	67.8	63.5
9	50.0	42.6	42.6	83.6	77.4	77.9
10	68.9	59.6	54.7	52.6	43.3	38.1
11	66.2	70.0	69.7	67.9	59.4	62.7

TABLE 8

SUMMARY OF DATA-GATHERING ITEMS SELECTED TO SOLVE
THE CASE PRESENTATIONS IN FOUR PROGRAMMED
EXAMINATIONS

Medical College of Georgia,
Junior Medical Students

	Experimental Group B' 3/12/65 N = 23	Control Group A' 4/30/65 N = 21
I. History Items		
L = Routine	64% of 1817	59% of 1659
M = Indicated	84% of 368	89% of 273
II. Physical Examination Items		
L = Routine	68% of 2438	48% of 2058
M = Indicated	86% of 1173	81% of 1239
III. Diagnostic Studies		
L = Routine	64% of 483	41% of 441
M = Indicated	60% of 1104	51% of 1071
N = Not Indicated	21% of 1403	16% of 1197
P = Contraindicated	23% of 184	25% of 189

During the course of the year, each student in each group worked his way through eight of these tests. Three were given as a pretest at the beginning of each clerkship, and five were given at the end as a post-test. The 100 students working through the eight tests made more than 100,000 clinical choices for us to evaluate and score. We have not yet completed the task. We do, however, have a tally of the choices made by the last experimental and control groups in the diagnostic sections of their four post-tests.

In their choices of history, physical, and especially of laboratory diagnostic items (table 8), the experimental group was consistently more thorough and somewhat more selective in their work-ups. In their performance in this written examination, they were consistently superior to the control group in every category. This is especially significant because this particular experimental group was relatively weak in its performance on the other written tests. In the other sections of the post-tests, dealing with formulations of diagnosis and specifications of plans for treatment, the experimental group generally made much better scores than did the control groups. The results of our written tests tend to support the findings of our oral examiners, but further analysis of the results and further study of the scoring systems will be necessary to be sure that the apparent differences represent valid differences in performance rather than artifacts of the test format or scoring system.

Summary

In our opinion, our study of the use of programmed materials for both the teaching and testing of patient-management skills has confirmed that this teaching method has great promise, but has also shown that the pitfalls in using this method are so numerous and the possibilities for errors in evaluation are so great that a final estimate of its value is not yet possible. We believe, though, that the phase of our project dealing with the evaluation of the "content" text demonstrates rather clearly that programmed materials, when compared with traditional methods of teaching, using conventional test methods as the measure of achievement, result in more efficient learning for the students and also permit more efficient use of faculty time.

References

1. McGuire, C. A. "Process Approach to the Construction and Analysis of Medical Examinations." *J. Med. Educ.* 38:556-563 (July) 1963.
2. Hubbard, J. P. and Clemans, V. *Multiple-Choice Examinations in Medicine—A Guide for Examiner and Examinee.* Philadelphia: Lea & Febiger, 1961.
3. Rimoldi, H. J. A. "Test of Diagnostic Skills." *J. Med. Educ.* 36:73-79 (January) 1961.

A Comparative Study of Lectures, Programmed Texts, and Programmed Films in Teaching Genetics to Medical Students

LUIS DAUFI*

A. FERNANDEZ-CRUZ**

THIS PAPER presents the results of an experiment designed to measure the relative effectiveness of three approaches to the teaching of genetics to third year medical students. While we were interested in a basic comparison of programmed and conventional methods of instruction, we were also interested in determining whether the accepted format of programming might be successfully replaced by a programmed "film" or television presentation. This latter approach would permit group instruction by means of the programmed material, and, in some circumstances, would be more compatible with conventional patterns of teaching than is a wholly individualized self-teaching treatment.

Design of the Study

Our procedure was to follow a simple, classic pattern of comparative treatment. Four groups of students were selected, three of which were distributed among the various instructional approaches while the fourth served as our control. A single achievement examination was given to all four groups at the same time. Examination scores served as a measure of effectiveness, and time spent by the

*Associate Professor
**Professor
Both of the Faculty of Medicine, The University of Barcelona, Spain.

7

Examinemos ahora de nuevo el núcleo celular interfásico del 2.

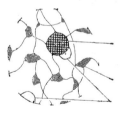

Si lo tratamos con clorhídrico para producir una hidrólisis parcial de los ácidos nucleicos y añadimos reactivo de Schiff, el núcleo queda teñido del siguiente modo:

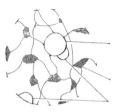

Vemos señalados los tres elementos que contienen nucleoproteínas.
a) Identifíquense de nuevo, escribiendo sus nombres junto al esquema.
b) ¿Qué estructura nuclear es negativa para la reacción de Feulgen?
....

8

Las desoxirribonucleoproteínas se destruyen específicamente por una enzima denominada **desoxirribonucleasa,** y las ribonucleoproteínas, por la **ribonucleasa.** Al tratar un corte de tejido con ribo- o desoxirribonucleasa, desaparece de la estructura celular la correspondiente nucleoproteína.

Así, un núcleo teñido con azán (colorante azul que se fija indistintamente sobre las nucleoproteínas) presenta el siguiente aspecto:

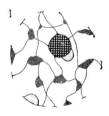

FIGURE 1

students in study was the measure of efficiency. Comparisons were made by means of statistical analysis and testing. Because we had no previous experience in the study of programmed learning, we constructed two null hypotheses anticipating no significant differences among the groups either in terms of effectiveness or efficiency.

The subjects were 118 third-year medical students. Their ages ranged from 20 to 22, and all had successfully completed their first two years of medical study, which includes courses in anatomy, biochemistry, histology, microbiology and psychology. All of them were now enrolled in a course in general pathology, a section of which is devoted to the particular study of genetics. All of the students were contacted by the experimenters and voluntarily agreed to take part in the study.

The groups were assigned at random, but modified in accordance with previous grade averages so that all of the groups were balanced in terms of known ability and achievement level.

Group A (n = 36) was assigned to the conventional lecture treatment. This was provided in the regular classroom according to usual procedures. They were allowed to take notes which could later be used for personal study. At the end of the lecture session, the students were given an opportunity to ask, and receive answers to, any questions that they wished. The students were urged to study the notes they had taken, and to consult any texts or other library materials they wish—with the proviso that they carefully record the time they actually spent on all forms of study.

Group B (n = 37) was assigned to the programmed teaching film protocol. The film was projected in their regular classrooms under lighting conditions which permitted the students to record notes as well as construct responses to the stimulus questions asked in the programmed film. The material was projected only once. No questions were answered, in keeping with the principle that the instructor was available only through the film medium. The students were permitted to study only their answer sheets and those other notes they had taken during the projection of the film. They were asked to record the time they spent in studying and to refrain from using other sources such as the library.

Group C(n = 34) received the programmed text. They were instructed to study only by means of this text and to record carefully the time they spent.

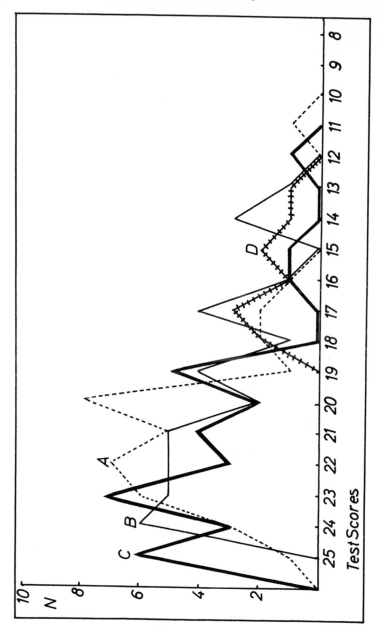

FIGURE 2

Group D (n = 11) received no instruction. This was our control group, intended to serve as a measure of pre-knowledge and general understanding.

Teaching Materials

The content of the first portion of the standard genetics text was included in the three instructional approaches. Specifically, the following areas were treated:

Composition of the cellular nucleus.
Ribonucleoproteins and desoxyribonucleoproteins.
The Feulgen reaction
Feulgen positive and Feulgen negative nuclear structures.
Contents of ribonucleoproteins in cytoplasm
Ergastoplasm, endoplasmic reticulum, ribosomes.
Function of the ribosomes.
Function of the endoplasmic reticulum.

group A Conventional Lecture		observed	adjusted
	N	36	35
	$S(x)$	746	735
mean	$\bar{x}$	20.7	21
	$S(x^2)$	15.717	15.596
variance	s^2	7.85	4.6
standard dev.	s	2.8	

TABLE 1

These subjects were not totally unknown to the students, for there had undoubtedly been references to some aspects of the content in previous courses, though not in considerable detail or in connected form. Precisely because we were not certain what the entering level of the students might be, we provided for Group D to help us eliminate the influence of prior instruction on achievement in the experimental groups.

The conventional lecture covered the materials listed above in a single session. The lecturer employed the blackboard and slide projections based on the illustrations used in the two programmed presentations. The time duration of the lecture was 45 minutes. The programmed text is a linear, Skinnerian sequence which covers the areas listed above in 20 frames. It was inexpensively printed and illustrated (a sample set of items is shown in figure 1). The programmed film is a direct audiovisual adaptation of the programmed text, and has a running time of 40 minutes.

group B Programed Lecture – Film		observed	adjusted
	N	37	
	$S(x)$	743	
mean	$\bar{x}$	20	20
	$S(x^2)$	15.832	
variance	s^2	30	
standard dev.	s	5.47	

TABLE 2

group C Programed Text		observed	adjusted
	N	34	
	S(x)	733	
mean	$\bar{x}$	21.5	21.5
	$S(x^2)$	16.120	
variance	s^2	20	
standard dev.	s	4.47	

TABLE 3

group D Control		observed	adjusted
	N	11	
	S(x)	160	
mean	$\bar{x}$	14.5	14.5
	$S(x^2)$	2.485	
variance	s^2	13.8	
standard dev.	s	3.71	

TABLE 4

Results and Analysis

One week after the various teaching protocols had been used, all of the students were given a 25 item objective examination of the multiple-choice type. The examination was designed to cover each of the areas included in the material; students were allowed 15 minutes to complete it. At the end of the test, the students were asked to record the time they had spent studying the material, aside from the original instruction. Scores and times were then subjected to statistical analysis.

The over-all results of the achievement test are graphically represented in figure 2. It can be observed, as was expected, that all of the experimental groups exceeded the achievement of the control group. Also, there is relatively little overlap in the curves, indicating that all of the forms of instruction accounted for gains in learning. Tables 1, 2, 3, and 4 show the statistical measures used to analyze the results. A test (table 5) for the significance of means confirms that all experimental groups were superior in achievement,

A B C D 21 20 21.5 14.5	A–B	A–C	B–D
degree of freedom	63	68	46
st. dev. dif. s_D	3.91	5.74	1.77
c	3.8	2.6	t 3.1
P	< 0.0001	< 0.01	< 0.01

TABLE 5

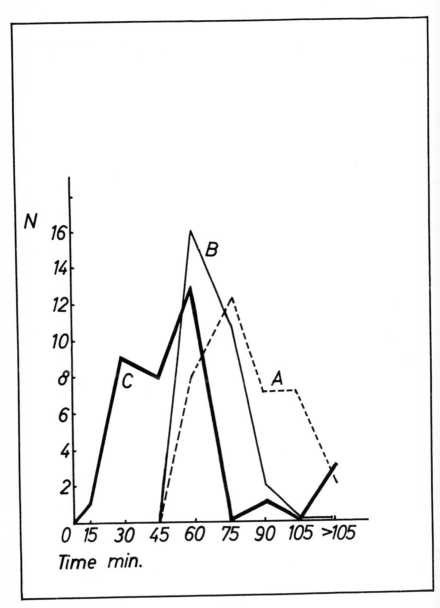

FIGURE 3

group A Conventional Lecture

TABLE 6		observed	adjusted
	N	36	35
	S(x)	3.045	2.820
mean	$\bar{x}$	84.5	80
	S(x²)	291.480	240.855
variance	s²	976	448
standard dev.	s	31.2	

group B Programed Lecture – Film

TABLE 7		observed	adjusted
	N	29	
	S(x)	1.736	
mean	$\bar{x}$	60	60
	S(x²)	106.830	
variance	s²	95.3	
standard dev.	s	9.74	

probability being below the .01 level. Likewise, a t-test for the significance of means indicates that the small score differences (group A, $\bar{x} = 21$; group B, $\bar{x} = 20$; group C, $\bar{x} = 21.5$) are statistically significant, largely due to the interaction of degrees of freedom and standard deviation, at the .05 level. While statistically significant, the quantitative difference is so slight that for practical, educational purposes, we feel it is more realistic to describe the three treatments as being equally effective.

In analyzing the time spent studying to arrive at a measure of efficiency, we included the times spent in the lecture by Group A and in the projection room by Group B. A distribution of the actual times is shown in figure 3. Observation of the curves shows clearly that there are some large differences, with the conventional lecture group taking most time and the programmed text group taking least. The differences between the means are all significant at below the .05 level, indicating that the programmed text is significantly more efficient. Tables 6, 7, 8, and 9 show the statistical measures used in arriving at results.

group C Programed Text		observed	adjusted
	N	34	33
	S(x)	1.830	1.680
mean	$\bar{x}$	53.8	50
	S(x²)	128.700	106.200
variance	s²	916	693
standard dev.	s	30.2	

TABLE 8

While this is only a beginning effort to develop and apply self-instructional methods, our findings substantiate that a learning program for medical students in genetics is as effective as conventional instruction and notably more efficient. Likewise, a self-instructional film employing techniques of programming proved to be as effective, and more efficient, than the lecture approach. If one were to construct a total performance index which included both the factors of efficiency and effectiveness, the programmed text would be the most favored teaching method, followed by the programmed film, this, in turn, followed by the lecture presentation.

Reactions of the students parallel the results of the methods, so that we have no hesitation in exploring further possibilities of self-instruction. One avenue that we certainly intend to study in more detail is that of programmed audiovisual techniques, which seem to be capable of results comparable to those obtained by the programmed text, and which permit class utilization as well as providing for some variation in presentation and treatment.

A B C 80 60 50	A–B	B–C
degree of freedom	63	67
st. dev. dif. s_D	5	4.9
c	4	2
P	< 0.0001	< 0.05

TABLE 9

Comparison of a Teaching Machine Program and a Series of Lectures in Electrocardiography

J. ANDERSON, M.B., D.S., MRCP*

S. G. OWEN, M.D., FRCP**

R. HALL, B.Sc., M.D., MRCP***

G. A. SMART, B.Sc., M.D., FRCP****

ALTHOUGH PROGRAMMED instruction has been shown to be an effective method of teaching in many fields, its applications to medical education have so far been limited, and few critical comparisons have been made between programmed and conventional materials. Our aim was to compare the efficiency and effectiveness of a program on electrocardiography presented by teaching machines, with that of a series of conventional lectures on the subject. The development of the program and a description of the validation process have been presented by Owen, Hall and Waller.[1, 2]

When two teaching methods are compared, several criteria must be borne in mind during the planning of the experiment. We were guided by the suggestions of Cheris.[3] The lectures were prepared from the machine program, thus providing two courses of identical content including the same concepts, examples, and illustrations.

*Lecturer in Medicine
**Senior Lecturer in Medicine and Academic Sub-Dean
***Wellcome Senior Research Fellow in Clinical Science
****Professor of Medicine
All from the University of Newcastle upon Tyne, England.

Considerable care was taken to ensure optimal quality of both presentations. Learning time was measured to assess the efficiency of each presentation, and the test used to measure effectiveness was designed to favor neither group.

Subjects

Seventy-seven medical students in their final year of study volunteered for participation in the trial. These students had little or no prior knowledge of electrocardiography. They were divided into two groups, matched on their results in previous professional examinations. An "academic rating" was derived by summing the marks obtained in these examinations. The mean ratings were identical (machine group 68.5, 19.52; lecture group 68.5, 20.59). There were, in the final experimental groups, 36 students studying the machine presentation and 41 attending the lectures. The discrepancy is due to the fact that several students asked to participate after the preliminary pairing had occurred. They were arbitrarily allocated to the lecture group because the number of machines was limited. Six female students were arbitrarily assigned to the machine group because, at the time, they were in a rotation at a maternity hospital and were unable to attend lectures. The academic rating was calculated on the basis of the final group arrangement.

Materials and methods

Electrocardiography is logical, self-contained, and well adapted for visual presentation, and therefore an appropriate subject for programming. The program was written by one of us (S. G. Owen) for the purpose of this trial. Prior to the trial, the program was "validated," i.e., tested, on a sample of the target population, in this case 12 final year medical students. As a result, the program was revised and in parts extended and rewritten. The final program* was of a branching type with some linear sequences, presenting both multiple-choice responding and constructional problems. It consisted of 604 pages or "frames," of which 254 represented the main sequence, the remainder containing remedial material.

The program was filmed on 35 mm film and presented by means of a Grundytutor teaching machine (International Tutor Machines, Ltd.). This presents the program by a rear projection device and is very similar in design and operation to the AutoTutor (U. S. Industries, Inc.)

*S. G. Owen, "Principles of Electrocardiography," International Tutor Machines, Ltd., Ashford, Middlesex, England.

The teaching machines were arranged in a large room in separate cubicles. Six were placed in the library of the maternity hospital for those students who were in residence there. In the main room 40 machines were available, permitting each student to have his or her own, with four reserve machines in case of breakdown.

The students were allowed to use the machines whenever they wished, and a technician was always available to deal with mechanical faults. During the three 50 minute periods each week, which corresponded to the lectures, one of us (J. A. Anderson) was in the room to provide general supervision. Each student was given a log-sheet on which to record the exact time he spent at the machine at each session.

The lectures were prepared from the program, and all examples and diagrams used were reproduced as slides from the program. Fourteen lectures, each of 50 minutes duration, were given by one of us (R. Hall). The number of lectures had not been fixed prior to the course, so that the lecturer could be allowed optimal coverage of the subject. A register was taken at each session; any students who missed lectures were contacted and the lecture was repeated to them before the next session.

All 77 students in the two groups completed the course within one month.

A few days after completion, teaching effectiveness was tested by means of a three hour examination in the theory and interpretation of electrocardiography. Multiple-choice questions were not used because the machine group were by then familiar with this technique, whereas the lecture group had had little experience with this type of problem.

The papers were identified by a code number and were scored independently in duplicate, according to a prearranged scheme. In the rare case of a discrepancy between marks, the paper was rescored jointly. Eight hospital residents and senior residents, four of whom had the assignment of reporting on the routine hospital electrocardiograms, took the same examination independently, to provide us with a reference standard.

In addition to the examination, the students were asked to complete a questionnaire designed to assess their reactions to the experiment. Specifically, the students in the machine group were asked their opinions of the machines, of the programs, and of this method

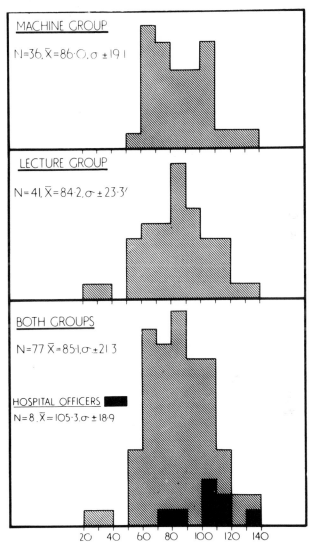

DISTRIBUTION OF SCORES IN FINAL ECG TEST

FIGURE 1

of learning. The lecture group was asked their opinions of the quality of the lectures and of the part they felt lectures played in the present medical curriculum. All students were asked to note the time they had spent on review of the subject outside the course, both during its administration and immediately prior to the examination.

Results and discussion

There was no significant difference betwen the mean scores on the final examination of the two groups (figure 1), and these scores compared favorably with those obtained by the eight hospital officers, confirming the effectiveness of both presentations.

The time taken to complete the teaching machine program (table 1) varied widely among the 36 students, the range being from 7 to 33 hours. The mean time was 14.3 hours ($\sigma = 5.82$). This was appreciably more than the 11.7 hours (fourteen 50-minute periods) spent in lecturing to the control group. However, the lecture group spent significantly more time on additional work during the course, so that the total learning time of the two groups was almost identical.

The difference between the times spent on additional work is presumably due to the continuous availability of the teaching machine for the program group of students. An appreciably smaller proportion of machine-taught students stated that they had taken systematic notes throughout the course (machine group 63.9 percent, lecture group 87.8 percent, $X^2 = 6.12; 0.025 > p > 0.01$).

There was no significant correlation between the final test score obtained and the total time spent in learning or the total additional time spent, nor were the mean scores higher for those who did extra work during the course than for those who did not. Immediate pre-examination review, however, did seem to be associated with a significant increase in performance ($p < 0.05$). Expression of the test scores as marks per unit of time spent in learning gives virtually identical "efficiency indices" for the groups.

The final test scores showed high correlation with the initial academic rating of the students ($r = +0.51, p < .001$).

This correlation was of importance for two reasons:

1. It was suggested that the matching procedure was reliable.
2. It permitted us to assess interaction effects between teaching method and other classifications such as sex or nationality, when analysis of covariance was applied to eliminate sampling fluctuations due to differences in initial academic ability.

TABLE 1

Learning Time and Efficiency Index

TEACHING METHOD

	Programmed	Conventional
Total learning time in hours, including all additional work	17.1	16.6
"Efficiency index" (test score per hour of learning time)	5.04	5.06

TABLE 2

Teaching Method in Relation to Previous
Academic Performance

TEACHING METHOD

Previous Academic Record	Programmed	Conventional
Group 1 (More than 1 S.D. above mean)	107.0	117.8
Group 2 (Between 0 and 1 S.D. above mean)	81.7	86.2
Group 3 (Between 0 and 1 S.D. below mean)	77.0	79.3
Group 4 (More than 1 S.D. below mean)	86.4	61.6
Interaction Variance p $<$ .10		

The interaction effect (table 2) between teaching method and academic ability may represent a meaningful trend ($.10 > p > .05$). This is largely due to the better performance of the machine-taught students in the lowest academic group (mean difference = 24.8, $t = 1.86, 0.10 > p > 0.05$).

Though the three higher groups show an increasing difference in favor of the lecture method, this trend does not reach statistical significance. Our results suggest, therefore, that for the academically weaker student, the teaching of electrocardiography by a machine program is more effective than learning from carefully prepared lectures.

Although there was no significant difference between the mean scores of the two sexes or between the two study groups as a whole, analysis of variance revealed a highly significant interaction effect between sex and teaching method (table 3).

The results suggested that men obtained more benefit from the machines, whereas women learned more effectively from the lectures. Analysis confirms the probability of both of these conclusions ($0.1 > p > 0.05$ and $0.05 > p > 0.02$ respectively).

Also, machine-taught men were probably superior to machine-taught women ($0.1 > p > 0.05$), although in the lecture group the women were superior to the men ($0.02 > p > 0.01$). Although this sex difference in teaching-method effectiveness was due in part to differences in initial academic ability among the subgroups, elimination of this bias by analysis of covariance reveals that there still appears to be a significant interaction between sex and teaching method.

One factor which may have contributed to this effect was the necessity for assigning six female students to the machine group because they were engaged in their resident maternity appointments. In relation to their known abiltiy, their performance in the test was lower than that of the other 71 students. This was no doubt due to the adverse factors which would tend to interfere with their effective studying, and the relatively low mean score in the female machine subgroup was presumably due in part at least to this experimental artifact.

Although there are few overseas students at Newcastle, it was felt important that their results be examined separately. Eleven of the 77 students who took part had a native tongue other than

TABLE 3

Teaching Method in Relation to Sex

TEACHING METHOD

	Programmed		Conventional		Totals	
	Mean	(Number)	Mean	(Number)	Mean	(Number)
Men	89.8	(24)	80.3	(33)	84.3	(57)
Women	78.3	(12)	100.4	(8)	87.2	(20)

Analysis of variance: Teaching method - not significant
                      Sex   - not significant
                                       - p $<$.01

TABLE 4

Teaching Method in Relation to
Overseas Students

TEACHING METHOD

ORIGIN		Programmed Mean		Conventional Mean		Totals Mean	
	Overseas	92.3	(4)	62.1	(7)	73.1	(11)
	British	85.2	(32)	88.8	(34)	87.0	(60)

(Figure in brackets refers to number)

English. The average performance of the overseas group was significantly lower than that of their British colleagues, even after covariance adjustment for their poorer previous academic record (table 4). It did not seem that this represented any special difficulty in electrocardiography, but rather that examiners consciously or subconsciously tend to make allowances for such handicaps as language difficulties. The E.C.G. test, being wholly objective, could not be so influenced, and thus the prior academic rating of the overseas students may be falsely high and the covariance adjustment not valid.

The overseas students in the machine group, however, performed as well as British students, while their colleagues in the lecture group appeared much worse. Correction for academic ability did not suggest that this finding was due entirely to chance (before covariance adjustment $p > 0.05$; after $p > 0.1$). As mentioned above, it is possible that within this group of students academic ratings were not valid and the poorer performance of the lecture group merely reflected their much poorer academic ability. The data do suggest, however, that these students are at a disadvantage when taught by conventional lectures, but this can be eliminated to some extent by programmed instruction.

Reactions of the students

The reaction, as judged by the questionnaire answers, was very favorable, toward both the program and the lectures. The students in the lecture group were almost unanimous in their praise of the high quality and excellent presentation of the lectures, and of the care which the lecturer had taken in preparing the subject. The responses of the machine students are shown in table 5. The majority felt that programmed instruction was more effective than conventional lectures, or textbooks, and again the majority felt that it was easier to concentrate on the machine program than on the other two. The main reasons for this positive feeling seems to be the motivation provided by the program. All but one student found the machine course to be motivating, and many were very enthusiastic about the challenge which they felt it presented. Some pointed out that the novelty of the method and the sense of competition engendered may, in part, have been responsible for this feeling of motivation.

Although major and minor mechanical breakdowns were not infrequent, they were rarely severe or sufficiently long-lasting to seriously interfere with a student's course of study. Some criticism

TABLE 5

Students' Reactions to Programmed Learning

	ANSWER	PERCENT
Do you think this method of learning is more or less effective than listening to lectures?	More	83
	Less	0
	About the same	11
	Not sure	6
Did you find it easier or harder to concentrate on the machine than you do on lectures?	Easier	69
	Harder	17
	About the same	14
	Not sure	0
Do you think this method of learning is more or less effective than reading the conventional textbook?	More	83
	Less	3
	About the same	11
	Not sure	3
Do you find it easier or harder to concentrate on the machine than you do on text-books?	Easier	75
	Harder	.6
	About the same	19
	Not sure	0

was expressed concerning the optical quality of the image and the operation of the focusing system. On the whole, however, the students found work with the machines efficient, pleasant and stimulating. Noise was perhaps the most common criticism, but did not seem to be more than a minor distraction to the majority of those who complained.

The students were asked for their opinion of the part that programmed instruction might be expected to play in medical education, and almost without exception they felt that it could have an important role. Some went so far as to say that this method could entirely replace conventional lectures. Diagnostic radiology, medical genetics and some aspects of clinical biochemistry were among the subjects which the students felt would lend themselves well to an effective programmed presentation.

Summary and conclusions

A comparison was made between a program presented by a teaching machine and a series of lectures, both offering identical content on electrocardiography to medical students. The students taking the program viewed it as motivating and well presented. The students attending the lectures felt they were of optimal quality and also felt they were well presented. The machine group students expressed their preference for this method over conventional methods of learning, and felt that programmed instruction could play an important part in the teaching of medicine.

Although no statistically significant difference was found by our study either in effectiveness or efficiency of the two teaching methods, we interpret this as a favorable result for the program, since few lecturers will have the benefit of a validated program from which to prepare their presentations, nor will they have the advantages which competition endows on themselves or their audience.

Our conclusions, after testing the knowledge acquired during our course, were that, for the circumstances here studied, programmed instruction:

1. Is probably more effective than conventional teaching for those whose native language is other than English.

2. Improves the performance of academically weaker students.

3. Is as effective as very carefully prepared lectures for students with average or good academic records.

4. May be more effective for male students.

5. Requires the same total learning time as conventional teaching.

ACKNOWLEDGEMENTS

The authors gratefully acknowledge the advice of Dr. J. L. Gibbons, M.D., D.P.M., MRCP, Senior Lecturer in Psychological Medicine; Mr. Duncan, Director of the University Department of Photography; and the technical assistance of Mr. and Mrs. R. Johnson.

References

1. Owen, S. G., Hall, R., and Waller, I. B. "Use of a Teaching Machine in Medical Education; Preliminary Experience with a Programme in Electrocardiography." *Post-grad. Med. J.,* 40:59-65 (February) 1964.

2. Owen, S. G., Hall, R., Anderson, J., and Smart, G. A. "Programmed Learning in Medical Education; An Experimental Comparison of Programmed Instruction by Teaching Machine with Conventional Lecturing in the Teaching of Electrocardiography to Final Year Medical Students." *Post-grad. Med. J.* 41:201-206 (April) 1965.

3. Cheris, B. H. On Comparing Programming and Other Teaching Methods. *J. Med. Educ.* 39:304-310 (March) 1964.

Part IV

Curricular Applications of Self-Instruction

Perhaps less glamorous than the tightly controlled research study, but quite as demanding, and just as necessary to our growth in understanding, is the field trial or extended use of self-instructional materials in the real-life teaching situation. Howard reports in droll form his experiences in teaching library skills. Lloyd discusses an investigation of student reaction to self-instructional courses. Garrett and Scott separately comment on programs designed for specific medical skills, while Garcia explains a large-scale curricular innovation that is beginning at California College of Medicine.

Self-Instruction in Using the Health Sciences Library: A Traveler's Tale

JOHN W. HOWARD*

FOREIGN TRAVELERS who see things differently than do the natives, and who then tell about the absurdities they met with, the wonders they saw, occupy a large place in literature. Of all such travelers, real and fictional, I have the greatest empathy with Mark Twain and his innocents. On their journey, you will remember, they were upon occasion amused, bewildered, confounded, filled with wondering approbation, and at last happy and a little astonished that they had survived.

I am such a foreign traveler, just such an innocent. I came to the land of self-instruction in medical education from the far-off country of the humanities. My immunization record was bare of courses in education. I had no booster shots of psychology. I knew almost nothing of the language of the place. The only natives I had met were Pipe's *Introduction to Dental Public Health: A Self-Instruction Course*[1] and Truelson's *How To Use a Medical Library*[2]. My only Baedecker was James L. Becker's *Programed Guide to Writing Auto-Instructional Programs*[3]. Traveling light, I was able to collect a number of souvenirs, and I would like to share some of them with you.

*Assistant Professor of Dental Literature, School of Dentistry, West Virginia University, Morgantown, West Virginia.

My journey really began two years ago, when the administration of the West Virginia University Medical Center decided—with complete justification—that our students needed instruction in the use of the library. As the result of a complex series of circumstances, I acquired the job of teaching the card catalog, using the traditional lecture-discussion format for each of the three groups into which the freshman medical and dental classes had been divided.

The effort required many, though uncounted, hours of preparation and 9 hours of classroom time for the teacher. An aggregate of about 600 hours of student time was spent. I regret to say that the course was not a triumph. The students had been asked—well, told—to give up most of their traditional between-semesters break, and they were in a mood that did not contribute noticeably to scholarly achievement. Now students who are merely acquiescent cannot disturb experienced teachers of composition; our psyches are too well keratinized for that. But I was disturbed. For one thing, I recognized my diminishing enthusiasm for the subject. If I did a reasonably good job on the Library of Congress classification scheme the first hour, the second presentation was certainly more cursory. The third time through, I let the class go early. Failing number one: the students did not receive equal instruction. Then a later group would raise a question on a matter which had been missed by an earlier group, and there was no chance to repair whatever harm had been done. Failing number two: course content could not be standardized among the various sections.

Quite clearly, something more radical than revision of my lecture notes was indicated. Just as clearly, the self-instruction approach offered a number of possibilities.

The first question I had to resolve was that of form. Should I use the vertical format? the horizontal? the fold-out answer sheet? My best answer was to use the scrambled text. It offered the greatest potential for satisfying my ideas of effective teaching.

I did not, of course, arrive at this decision without trying the other forms, all of which I found objectionable for one reason or another. In the vertical format, for instance, I found myself cheating. The paper covering the answers would slip down, I would read the correct answers, and the carefully prepared self-instruction text was quickly metamorphosed into an ordinary textbook. No matter how effective the text might be as a self-instruction program, it was repetitious, primerlike, and dull when used as a simple text. Call it a lack of moral fiber if you will, call it a perversion of the whole idea of self-instruction; the fact remains that the vertical format and I simply did not get along well together. The other linear formats didn't enchant me, either. True, I couldn't cheat as easily, but I soon felt the endless drip-drip-drip of information was close kin to that water torture the Chinese are supposed to have designed. My feeling for the scrambled text is best explained in terms of a statement that I didn't run across until much later. A physician is recalling his days in medical school:

> The light was dim, the whole place dusty and littered with cigarette stubs and matches, the air so hot and foul that frequently students fainted . . . Eight hours of this on hard benches . . . Cat calls, whistles and yells greeted the Professor and often interrupted his lecture . . . The lecture was given in the precise and deadly manner common at the time. The steady voice droned on hour after hour in bald scientific statements with not a gleam of spirit or a hint of humor.[4]

As it happens, he was reminiscing about student life nearly a hundred years ago. His objections are still relevant.

I wanted to avoid being a drone. I wanted to be precise, but not deadly. For a noncredit course in a subject that students regard as extraneous to their education, I felt that a gleam of spirit, perhaps a hint of humor, would not be misplaced. These were all compatible with the scrambled text.

I prepared such a text. It has been used by one class of freshman medical students, and copies have been circulated for review among members of the Medical Library Association. Its use and the comments made about it have given me the same emotions Mark Twain noted: I have been variously amused, bewildered, confused, and filled with approbation. I am happy and a little astonished that I survived as well as I have.

Many of the ingredients in my mixture of emotions came from the librarians. I hadn't expected their responses to be so contradictory. One librarian wrote, "Use of the scrambled text, especially in a text this long, will discourage potential users from ever completely reading the text." Another gave rather a dubious blessing: "The novelty value of a scrambled book will likely persuade many students to go through the whole book—or at least much of it." Still a third librarian was most generous; he wrote, "For a change I found a book describing library procedures in a way not guaranteed to produce a fit of sleeping sickness. I was quite pleased and I should think that a student would be hard put whether to finish [reading] *Candy* or devote his time to the decipherment of catalog procedures."

The librarians were divided about self-instruction techniques, too. Said one, "I don't believe the method will take the place of the good old-fashioned lecture in education. It takes too long to get to the next point using the 'programmed' approach." To the contrary, another remarked, "This type of learning is being used more and more by schools, so I think this will have a place in the curriculum . . . Already the 'scrambled text' is being used for more difficult subjects, e.g., how to read an electrocradiogram, so why not the card catalog?"

Some librarians were offended because I was—these were their terms—"elementary," "juvenile," and "chatty." "The book," wrote one, "lacks dignity and value as a teaching guide." Others were more complimentary; one of this group said "Meat of the matter is excellent—clear, sufficiently detailed and sufficiently concise, directed to the user."

Finally, one librarian reported that her staff feels the book is "aimed at a college freshman rather than at a higher level." On this point, another commented, "We feel that the text is too difficult to handle and that this type of instruction would not be beneficial to students below the graduate level."

I'll not try to assign to these quotations the emotion that each evoked. When the time comes to revise the work, I won't pay very much attention to them, either. But I shall pay considerable attention to the comments of the students who used the text. It was, after all, aimed at them.

Briefly, the situation was this: The books were distributed after a minimum amount of orientation. The students were dismissed to work at their own speed for the remainder of the week. Total teacher's time elapsed, ten minutes. At the week's end, we met again to discuss the material and to fill out a questionnaire. Total teacher's time now elapsed, one hour. Remember, I had spent three hours with each group the previous year. With the self-instruction text, the teacher's time was reduced by two thirds.

The students were asked to comment on programmed instruction. Some didn't like it at all, while others found it a completely satisfactory way to learn. Perhaps the most unabashedly honest comment, and certainly one of the most satisfying notes, came from a student who wrote "It was an enjoyable book, considering that I am not interested in the subject."

The questionnaire elicited the information that 34.6% of this group of freshman medical students claimed previous experience with programmed teaching. I trust the remaining 65.4% were not prejudiced against self-instruction techniques by their first meeting with it. I don't believe they were, for the questionnaire asked them to record their general reaction to this type of teaching, and the results came out like this:

Highly opposed	2%
Opposed	4%
Neutral	22%
Favorable	58%
Highly favorable	10%

The students were also asked to note the amount of time they had spent on the text. Of those who responded, these were the results:

½ hour	8.3%
¾ hour	8.3%
1 hour	25.0%
1¼ hours	4.2%
1½ hours	39.6%

Here also was real time saving. Traditional classroom procedures had required three hours from each student. Self-instruction techniques reduced this to an average of slightly more than 1¼ hours, or less than half the time needed for the lecture-discussion approach.

All this was very well. My time had been saved. The students' time had been saved. A clear majority of the students found self-instruction a satisfactory way to learn. But had they, in fact, learned?

Yes, they had. An objective pre-instruction test on the choice of subject headings (the most difficult part of using the card catalog) showing a median score of 56 percent. A similar post-instruction test showed a median score of 69 percent. This is a gain in median score of nearly 25 percent, a gain which a friend in our College of Education says I can call "very adequate."

These, then, are some of the notes and snapshots I took on my first journey through the land of self-instruction. It was not a long-lasting trip, but it was for the most part an enjoyable one. Certainly I learned a great deal, and for that reason, if for no other, I believe the trip was rather successful. And while I would hate to be classified as one of those tourists who became an expert on the Irish question because his jet had a one-hour layover at Shannon airport, I do feel bound to conclude with some of my reactions to, and generalizations about, this unfamiliar land I have visited.

First, I am delighted that students took so well to what was a new form of learning for most of them, and that they learned so well from it. It's probably best merely to be grateful for good student motivation, without probing too deeply into their reasons for learning without a teacher in residence. To do so is to run quickly into the notion that when the student's mood or the circumstances of the moment are somehow inappropriate to learning, it is far easier to close a book than it is to shut up a living, breathing teacher.

Second, I am impressed by the saving of time and the standardization of course content that self-instruction techniques afford. I don't know to what uses students might put the hours that would be saved if all their education could be so considerably shortened, but I do know a great many ways in which I could use the time now spent in the classroom. Standardization has its uses, too. With reasonable attention on his part, each student would be exposed to exactly the same material. Putting this and other obvious advantages aside, we would no longer have people like that apocryphal naval cadet who dropped his pencil during a lecture on naval history and missed the whole Civil War, or that medical student who missed a lecture in microbiology and now believes that viruses were invented by someone who couldn't spell gastroenteritis.

Finally, I am convinced that the scrambled text is the most efficacious of the self-instruction forms. A kind of controlled Socratic dialog, it has particular advantages for those learning episodes in which judgment and decision are as important as accumulation and response—in those educational areas, that is to say, that we call "art" when we speak of the "art and science" of a field. Regardless of the situation in which it might be used, the scrambled text adds to the virtues of any self-instruction method one more than is uniquely its own; a sense of persons. By this, I mean two things. There is, first a semblance of student-teacher contact, the lack of which has been central to the widespread disquiet and rebellion we have recently seen in college students. I see no reason to believe that medical schools are immune to this rebellion, though to my knowledge they have so far escaped the infection. But would it not be wise in the use of self-instruction material to apply the preventive measure of a 1:1 student-teacher ratio? This the scrambled text can do. Second, the sense of person which the scrambled text offers to the student applies as well to the teacher. Has any outstanding teacher been other than a strong personality? Has he not had unlimited enthusiasm, and has not that enthusiasm been conveyed almost synaptically to his students? Such enthusiastic personalism is native to the scrambled text alone. It is my favorite region in the land of self-instruction. I commend it to your use.

References

1. Pipe, Peter. *Introduction to Dental Public Health: A Self-Instruction Course.* San Francisco: U. S. Department of Health, Education and Welfare, Public Health Service, Division of Dental Public Health and Resources, Dental Health Center, 1964.
2. Truelson, Stanley, D., Jr. *How to Search the Medical Literature.* Rochester, New York: The University of Rochester Medical Library, 1964.
3. Becker, James L. *A Programmed Guide to Writing Auto-instructional Programs.* Camden: RCA Educational Programs, 1963.
4. Gardiner, C. F. "Getting A Medical Education in New York City in the Eighteen-seventies." (Cited in Annan, Gertrude L., "Medical Americana" *J.A.M.A.,* 195:131-136, 1965.)

Student Reactions to
Self-Instructional Materials

JOHN S. LLOYD*

THIS IS A REPORT of our experiences in seeking medical student reactions to three units of self-instructional materials. These reactions were obtained with a structured interview in which a prepared list of questions was asked of all the students. The self-instructional materials were of the clinical case-problem variety, and were developed for the instruction of second-year medical students on three separate topics. These were: tumors of the lung, the red blood cell, and disorders of the gastrointestinal tract. The materials were "self-instructional" in the sense that they were designed to guide and encourage self-education in the student's free time.

This paper will describe those three self-instructional units and the method used to collect student reactions to them. Some over-all impressions of student responses to this project will be presented, along with an interpretation of those student reactions thought to be of general interest, particularly those which involve comparisons between the different teaching methods. Finally, some comments will be made about the value of student reactions in the evaluation of educational methods.

Description of self-instructional materials
Tumors of the Lung: Each student was given a folder contain-

*Research Assistant, Division of Research in Medical Education, Western Reserve University School of Medicine.

ing the self-instructional materials, comprised of six actual cases involving intrathoracic neoplasms, in the form of paper and pencil tasks. Each problem contained a written case history, physical examination, laboratory findings, and photographic reproductions of radiologic and histologic specimens, all taken from cases in the files of University Hospitals of Cleveland. The photographic reproductions of x-rays were black and white, glossy photoprints on 8½" x 11" stock; the histologic reproductions were 35 mm Kodachrome transparency slides. These slides contained gross and microscopic views of the various lesions represented. (Slide viewers were made available to the students on loan.)

In the course of working through a case problem, the student was required to read a segment of clinical data and then respond to specific questions regarding the data. Immediately after responding, the student could turn the page and find the correct answers. Next, the student was provided with further information about the patient and was then asked to respond to several more questions. By proceeding to the next page, he could compare his response with the correct answers. This was continued for each case, until the student reached a diagnosis and prescribed the treatment. The materials were thus presented somewhat in the fashion of programmed workbooks, allowing the student to progress in a stepwise manner, obtaining immediate feedback to his responses.

Gastrointestinal Diseases: Here each student was presented with seven case problems, each on a different disorder. Again the written case histories, physical examination, and laboratory findings were supplemented by photographic reproductions of radiologic and histologic specimens. With this unit the reproductions were all black and white, glossy photoprints of varying sizes: 35 mm Kodachrome slides were not used. Unlike the programmed workbook format of the lung tumor materials outlined above, the gastrointestinal case problems presented the student at once with *all* the information necessary for a diagnosis.

The student was asked several questions about *all* the data rather than specific questions about parts of it. In addition, the answers to these general questions were not provided on succeeding pages, but were distributed at a later date, thus providing delayed rather than immediate feedback to the student.

The Red Blood Cell: During the past few years, the School of

Medicine at Western Reserve University has been one of several schools participating in a cooperative research endeavor to evaluate a method of teaching hematology—a method emphasizing self-education. A more detailed explanation of this research project can be found in articles by Harris, *et. al.*[1], and Ginther[2].

In general, the purpose of the project has been to compare two methods of teaching about the red cell: one employing the traditional didactic triad of lectures, laboratories, and readings from a syllabus[3]; the other employing small group discussions, patient presentations, and a self-instructional workbook (unillustrated) of clinical case problems[4], in addition to laboratories and syllabus—but no lectures.* The two methods have been evaluated by comparing the objective test performance of those students taught by the traditional or "control" method in one group of medical schools, with the performance of other students taught by the "experimental" methods in a second group of medical schools.

Until the past year the School of Medicine at Western Reserve University has been among those schools employing the "experimental" method. Last year, however, it was decided that all the schools would exchange protocols—that for the first half of the teaching unit, the "control" schools would become "experimental," and vice versa. For the second half of the teaching unit the schools could adopt whichever method they preferred. Therefore, this past year the School of Medicine of Western Reserve University taught the first half of the red cell unit in the "control" manner and the second half in the "experimental" manner, providing an opportunity for study of the two methods almost side by side.

Description of structured interview method

A climate has been fostered at this school of medicine which encourages student participation in educational planning and evaluation. In keeping with this approach, student reactions to the teaching methods were sought. The materials on lung tumors and gastrointestinal diseases were being employed for the first time and it was judged desirable that student views concerning the value of the materials and suggestions for improvements should be sought immediately. As all three units were intended to encourage students to take responsibility for educating themselves, we also sought to learn how they actually went about using the materials. Finally, the de-

*This was the original format of the project. This past year, however, for reasons of the research design, lectures were included.

sign of the hematology project provided a unique opportunity for students to make direct inter-method comparisons.

Several considerations led to the selection of the structured interview as the method for collecting students' responses. The chief alternative to the interview as a data-gathering instrument is the questionnaire. While the questionnaire can provide an investigator with quantitative data from a large sample of subjects, it was felt for our purposes that information in depth from a small, random sample was more useful. The interview provides an opportunity for asking questions which encourage a fuller response than a simple "yes" or "no" (or a check mark in a box); moreover, the interview permits the investigator to ask the student to expand on particular responses. As this was our initial attempt at collecting reactions to these particular materials, we had many questions to ask the students. We felt that a lengthy questionnaire might well be perceived by the students as just another form to fill out and, consequently, one to be disregarded or given little thought. In contrast the interview permits the investigator to ask many detailed questions, at the same time establishing rapport with individual students and emphasizing the importance of their opinions in the eyes of the faculty.

A list of questions to be asked was devised with the help of the faculty members concerned. The questions were edited so as not to suggest responses to the students, and pretested for clarity and appropriateness. The questions were then used as a guide by the interviewer, the standardized list providing some consistency in the stimuli presented to each student.

Some general categories of questions asked in the interviews were: How much time did the students spend with these self-instructional materials? What use did students make of the answers that were immediately available in the programmed workbooks? From which materials did the students think they learned more, and which materials did they prefer? What was their over-all opinion concerning each unit of self-instructional materials, and what improvements would they suggest for each unit? Where appropriate, the students were queried about lectures, laboratories, discussions, and other aspects of the curriculum.

Because the case problems on lung tumors were presented earlier in the year than were the gastrointestinal and hematology materials, two sets of interviews were conducted with two random samples of

10 students each. From samples of this size it was felt that the results could be generalized to a population the size of one medical school class (N = 79).

A carefully written letter was sent to the students in both samples explaining the purpose of the interview and requesting their cooperation. Shortly after receiving this letter, each student was contacted by telephone and an appointment for an interview was made. All interviews were conducted by the same investigator, and each interview was tape-recorded with the permission of the student. The responses to each question were then transcribed, and a tabulation was made of the frequency of each response to each question.

Because the students' reactions collected by means of these interviews are qualitative in nature, because the interviews were conducted some time after the students had used the materials and therefore relied heavily on the students' memories, and because the data were analyzed by only one person—the interviewer—the interpretations must be seen as impressionistic. With this caution in mind, let us proceed to a few interpretations which may be of general interest.

Some impressions and interpretations

The students appeared to welcome the opportunity to participate in this evaluation of the materials they had used. One indication of this was that all 20 selected students accepted the invitation to participate in the interviews. Generally, the students praised the faculty for attempting new methods of presenting subject matter, and expressed their desire to have more areas taught in a similar manner. Their over-all opinion of the self-instructional materials was very favorable. This halo of enthusiasm, however, did not blunt the students' critical comments concerning some aspects of the materials, and the ways they were presented. The students' criticisms were uniformly offered in a constructive vein and appeared to be based on well-considered reasons.

One advantage of the interview method is that it permits the interviewer to probe for reasons behind reactions. The students underscored this general response by pointing out that there were two basic reasons for their favorable reaction to these self-instructional materials: first, the materials were indeed self-instructional, and did succeed in shifting the responsibility for learning to the students; and second, the students felt a genuine sense of accomplishment from being able to work with, and solve, realistic medical problems. The students felt a strong need for realism—they wanted to feel like physicians, solving realistic medical problems, and using their own resources.

This apparent need for realism was manifested in at least two ways. The first became evident when the students were asked to compare the "experimental" half of the hematology course, which employed immediate feedback, with the gastrointestinal disorders unit which employed delayed feedback. Nine out of ten students chose the method using *delayed* feedback as being both more effective and personally preferred.

There are several possible reasons for this choice. The gastrointestinal cases were purposely selected to represent *typical* disease problems, whereas the hematology cases were chosen because they were unusual. The students may have found the typical cases easier to diagnose. The gastrointestinal cases employed photographs to illustrate radiologic and histologic evidence, whereas in the hematology workbook there were no illustrations. But the overwhelming reason given was that the delayed feedback of the gastrointestinal materials provided a closer simulation of reality than did the immediate feedback of the hematology materials.

While the step-by-step manner of the hematology materials provided a prototype of an organized approach to the diagnosis of disease (the value of which the students recognized), the students found these materials somewhat artificial. They called for isolated facts rather than an understanding of the subject matter; and the correct answers were on the next page—which is not the case in medical practice.

On the other hand, the gastrointestinal materials with delayed feedback required a more advanced, professional approach. Students had to search for their own answers; they could see greater interrelationships of facts and could perceive the way these facts contributed to the final diagnosis and treatment.

The second instance of the students' need for realism occurred in their responses to questions regarding the use of 35 mm Kodachrome slides in association with the unit on tumors of the lung. Photographic slides had been used for the following reasons:

1) In contrast to regular glass tissue slides, 35 mm slides allowed an identical gross or microscopic view of a lesion to

be made available to all students in the class, even at different times.

2) The 35 mm slides were not restricted to the laboratory. They could be taken along with the other materials, to each student's usual place of study, so that all necessary data for a diagnosis would be readily at hand.

3) After the student finished using the 35 mm slides, they could be stored with the other materials for future reference.

4) While photoprints would have been preferred, as reproductions, the cost of processing such a small quantity of color photographs would have been prohibitive.

Unexpectedly, the students objected to the 35 mm slides. One of the most frequently stated reasons was that they preferred to acquire the experience of looking at regular glass tissue slides through a microscope because this is what they would have to do in arriving at a real diagnosis. Furthermore, the microscope allows the student to view the lesion at different magnifications and search out the abnormal tissue in the specimen (as he would have to do in reality) rather than having the abnormal tissue clearly identified by the 35 mm slide.

When students were asked to compare the two teaching methods used in the hematology course—the one using the traditional didactic method and the other employing, among other things, a programmed workbook format—they overwhelmingly endorsed the second approach. In addition to exhibiting again the need for realism described above, the reasons given for the choice of the second approach also seemed to reveal the students' need for structure. The syllabus[3] used is notoriously esoteric, covering the red cell in wide scope, and displaying considerable depth as well as breadth. Many view it as a complete reference work on the red cell. Yet, under the traditional method, the students were assigned large portions of this syllabus. In the words of one student, the material to be learned was "just . . . dumped on us and we were supposed to sort it out ourselves." In the "experimental" approach the addition of the case problem workbook and the accompanying small group discussions helped the students ferret out the important aspects of the syllabus—something they felt was missing in the traditional method. Having to work through actual cases on their own apparently helped the students to structure the mass of factual material with which they were confronted.

Although comparisons were not made among *all three* units of materials, spontaneous comments made by the students in the course of the interviews seem to indicate that the *newer* materials involving lung tumors and gastrointestinal disorders were preferred to the relatively older hematology problems. Again, a number of things could account for this preference, but the students' comments strongly suggest that this is not exclusively a function of the *materials* themselves. Rather, it appears that this preference for the newer case problems in part reflects the attitudes of the faculty. That is, because the lung tumor and gastrointestinal materials were also new to the faculty, they may have been introduced with a great deal of enthusiasm which radiated to the students. On the other hand, several years of use may have somewhat diminished the enthusiasm with which the hematology faculty presented its materials, at least as it was perceived by the students.

Finally, since the correct answers were provided immediately in the lung tumor and red cell workbooks, and since these materials were designed for the students to use on their own time in their own study areas, we inquired as to the use students made of the answers provided. We wanted to know whether students actually committed themselves to writing a response prior to consulting the correct answer (the manner in which the materials were intended to be used), or if they used the workbooks more as textbooks, merely reading the answers without first attempting to write a response.

The majority of the students indicated that they used the materials in the desired manner because they felt that only in this way would they derive the maximum benefit from the materials. Of those who looked at the correct answers without responding in writing, some said they attempted to formulate a response in their minds before looking at the answers. The main reason given for not writing down a response was pressure of time. Most of these students felt that the amount of time they could afford to spend working through the case problems was not sufficient to permit a written response.

These have been just a few of the impressions derived from our experience in gathering student reactions to self-instructional materials. It is anticipated that the verbatim responses of the students will be of some value as guidelines for the faculty in planning for the future.

Student reactions and the evalution of teaching methods

In the evaluation of educational innovations, such as the three units of self-instructional materials outlined above, the main issue usually has been whether or not these newer teaching methods, when contrasted with other teaching methods, enhance the learning of the subject matter. Relatively little attention has been paid to the systematic collection of student opinion regarding the newer teaching methods and, especially when self-instructional materials are involved, learning just how students go about using these materials. When student opinion has been surveyed in the past, it has usually been as a by-product of the search for achievement.

I submit that student reactions and opinions are important in their own right, and that their effect on the learning process may be of some consequence. Most of us would agree that learning is partly a function of the motivation to learn, and partly a function of *how* one learns. At this point, the relationship between the responses of students in these interviews and their actual learning of the subject matter in the courses employing self-instructional materials can only be conjectured. For example, did the students who responded in writing before looking at the answers in the programmed workbooks learn more from these materials than those who did not? Behavioral theory would generally predict that overt responding prior to reinforcement enhances learning. But does this relationship hold up in practice?

Another interesting question is: do those students who specify one particular teaching method as being more effective actually learn more from the method of their choice? For example, do those students who prefer a delayed feedback format actually learn more from this method than do those students who prefer an immediate feedback format, and vice versa?

The theory behind programmed instruction would predict that most people learn better from an immediate feedback format. It may be, however, that the nature of clinical case problems makes them more effective in a delayed feedback format. While these questions remain to be answered by empirical evidence, it may well be that there is no *one* best teaching method for all students, and that only out of a variety of teaching methods from which students can choose will there accrue the greatest learning for the greatest number.

References

1. Harris, J. W., D. L. Horrigan, J. R. Ginther and T. H. Ham. "Pilot Study in Teaching Hematology, with Emphasis on Self-Education By the Students." *J. Med. Educ.* 37:719-36 (August) 1962.

2. Ginther, J. R. "Cooperative Research in Medical Education: An Example From Hematology." *J. Med. Educ.* 38:718-24 (September) 1963.

3. Harris, J. W. *The Red Cell: Production, Metabolism, Destruction: Normal and Abnormal.* Cambridge, Massachusetts: Harvard University Press, 1963.

4. Harris, J. W. and D. L. Horrigan. *Case Development Problems in Hematology: Series 1: The Red Cell, Problems 1-8.* Cambridge, Massachusetts: Harvard University Press, 1963.

A Modified Programmed Presentation of Neuroanatomy

FREDERIC D. GARRETT, Ph.D.*

IN DISCUSSING the ideal form for presenting a medical course, Cheris has written, "Perhaps the best solution would be to combine the most favorable qualities of both the program and the text, that is, employ the conciseness and continuity of a text and the active student participation and self-testing required by a program."[1] This paper reports the gradual evolution over 5 years of just such an approach to the presentation of a 100-hour medical course in neuroanatomy at the University of Miami School of Medicine.

History of the project

A problem arose in 1960. We noted a sharp fall in student performance which appeared to be caused by at least two factors. We were still dealing with "depression babies"—scraping the bottom of the barrel for qualified applicants. Superimposed on this was an administrative edict reducing the preliminary examinations in the course from five to one. This not only deprived the students of the disciplinary goad; it also deprived them of an essential guide to, and measure of, accomplishment. A programmed presentation suggested itself as the possible remedy for both deficiencies.

In 1961 a rather conventional branching program, following the sequence of topics presented in the reference text, was prepared for a small segment of the course, and in 1962 it was extended to the

*University of Miami School of Medicine

whole course. It then became apparent that the sequence of topics was not sufficiently systematic and that the branching form was unsuited to the large presentation. Over a small area it intrigued the student, but over a whole subject it became monotonous and obscured the important concepts with details.

So, in 1963 an independent program was prepared. This was in linear form, but unconventional in that it contained much paragraphed information, and less step-by-step leading than the usual program. This modification was made necessary by the fact that the conventional small-step form would create a unit so bulky that the student could not even read it in the time available.

This hastily written and highly imperfect 1963 program was thoroughly revised in 1964. With incidental imperfections removed it was possible to see the need for further major alterations, which led to the current (1965) version. This is, essentially, a highly structured text combined with provision for student response and feedback on correctness, and it appears to meet the specifications in the quotation from Cheris.

Description of the program

The 1962, 1963 and 1964 versions attempted to cover the entire course in neuroanatomy, a larger field than has been attempted in most previous programs. The major alteration in the present version was to sort out something like 30 to 40 percent of the concepts as being truly vital, and to include only these in the main presentation. The excluded concepts will be presented in abbreviated form in a supplementary program. The vital concepts are bundled into 142 unitary presentations which we call "sets."

In each set, text and questions are physically separated (figure 1). The textual material is often presented in outline rather than paragraphs, and illustrated with simple diagrams. Many directions of the form, "Now do thus and so," are included. Most of the concepts are extremely simplified and qualifying statements are held to a minimum. The length of the text in a given set is determined entirely by the requirements of its subject, ranging from 7 to 850 words with a mean of around 225 words.

Questions in each set are placed after the text, with answers printed beside the question in the left margin so that they can be covered with a card, but can then be checked immediately and with a minimum of effort. Many students are convinced that they pro-

4.

CHAPTER I. FUNDAMENTALS.

<u>Set 1. The basic concept</u>.

<u>Sensation</u> leads to <u>behavior</u> through interconnections provided by the nervous structures (as represented semi-humorously in fig. 1):

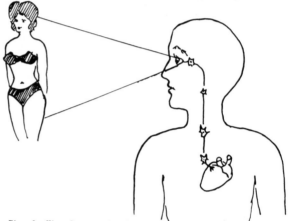

Fig. 1. Visual sensation leading to behavior (increased heart rate).

<u>Sensation</u> (as used here) is the activity of sense organs, called <u>receptors</u> (eye in fig. 1). Receptor activity arises from <u>stimuli</u> which fall upon the organ. A <u>stimulus</u> is some change occurring in the conditions surrounding the body or within it. (But a change becomes a stimulus only if some part of the body responds to it— is sensitive to it, as we usually say.)

<u>Behavior</u> is the sum-total of movements resulting from activity of <u>effector</u> organs, that is, muscles and glands (cardiac muscle in fig. 1). Significant behavior adjusts the organism in some appropriate way to the environmental conditions which have evoked the behavior-promoting sensation (increased blood pressure in fig. 1).

Receptor.   So, the sequence of events is: stimulus; activity of _____;
Effector.   activity of nervous structures; activity of _____; movement
               (of a part of the body or of some substance within it).

FIGURE 1

gress most rapidly by studying the question together with the uncovered answer.

The program is squarely based on the principle of proceeding from the general to the specific. It commences with the simplest statement one can make concerning the over-all significance of the nervous system (figure 2) and endeavors to proceed from this in such a way that the student never loses sight of how the material under consideration at the moment fits into the total picture.

Observations

We have experienced one conspicuous adverse result. Students, while learning more, have been less happy with the course than in pre-program days. Although there is considerable overt praise of the program, and little overt criticism, there is almost none of the spontaneous enthusiasm which students displayed toward the course outline which the program replaced. Also, the class shows less tendency to go back over the early part of the course when preparing for examinations. Review not specifically incorporated in the program tends to be neglected.

Favorable results, however, are so preponderant that I cannot imagine willingly returning to a non-programmed presentation. Grade curves for the five years involved are displayed in the table (figure 3). It is impossible to say just what these mean because program effects are confounded with other factors—especially the fact that average capacity of the student body has increased as the war babies have arrived, giving the admissions committee more from whom to choose. It is apparent from direct observation of the class, however, that the program has produced a definite change in the level of learning. Students master the fundamentals both earlier and better, and then go on to worry about more advanced topics, which former classes largely ignored.

From the viewpoint of the teaching staff, the biggest advantage of the program is that the course is now easier to administer. Most medical students consider neuroanatomy the most difficult first-year subject. This is due partly to its innate complexity, but chiefly to the student's total unfamiliarity with the concepts and the pyramidal structure of these concepts. If early concepts are not mastered, later ones are not intelligible. In the past, administering the course has been a constant battle to keep the class from lagging so far behind that current presentations became ineffective. With the program,

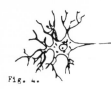

Axon

8.

Fig. 4.

Ten.

Thought question:

Given 10 sense cells and 10 effector cells, what minimum number of separate neuron chains would be necessary to transfer the sensory pattern to the effector cells with no loss or alteration?

Note - This kind of simple one to one relationship between receptor and effector cells exists only in a few special situations.

Set 5. Form of the neuron (figs. 4 and 5):

Large, rounded, nucleus-containing central portion-- the **cell body** or **perikaryon** ("karyon", pronounced "carry on", refers to the nucleus).

Extending outward from the cell body are slender thread-like processes of two kinds-- **axons** and **dendrites** ("dendron" is greek for "tree". Note the tree-like branching).

Axons usually extend out to great distances (fig. 4), and establish **synaptic contact** with other neurons (or effector cells). They constitute the essential part of the **nerve fiber**.

Typical **dendrites** are relatively short and highly branched. They provide increased surface area for receiving synaptic contact from incoming axons.

Axon

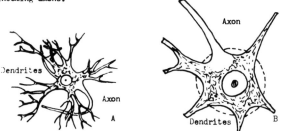

Dendrites

Axon

A

Axon

Dendrites

B

Fig. 5. Cell structure of neuron.

Cell body, axon, dendrite.   What are the three major parts of the neuron?

Axon.   Which kind of process is wire-like?

Axon.   Which process represents the nerve fiber?

To synapse
or effector cell

FIGURE 2

this problem has largely disappeared. Many students study ahead of the class schedule, providing a marked increase in their receptivity to the classroom presentation.

Possibly the greatest satisfaction in administering a program lies in the instructor's confidence that the concepts are being placed before the class fully and with balanced emphasis. Theoretically this should be accomplished by the conventional textbook. In practice, however, most medical students define as important only what they hear in lecture. It appears that they extend this definition to include the content of the program.

Discussion

We feel that in our hands the program has demonstrated its superiority over the class outline in teaching a complex subject to a group of medical students.

Medical teaching must proceed under conditions determined by the need for a tremendous mass of information to be absorbed in far too little time. The lower half of the class, at least, seems pressed to work to the very limits of their capacity. Injudicious study habits develop. Sleep and food are neglected. Anxiety, if not panic, easily takes root and sweeps the class.

Under these conditions the student will not tolerate anything which adds to the mechanical bulk of his work. He is intensely motivated and highly capable of absorbing masses of information in condensed form. He insists on knowing where he is going and why.

The conventional short-step program generally fails to meet these requirements in several ways:

1. It takes too much time.

2. It submerges the student in details from which the generalizations emerge, if at all, too slowly and with insufficient clarity.

3. It does not provide an outline of the conceptual structure of the subject. It is almost impossible to skim the conventional program for either preview or review. The student is not kept continually oriented as to what he is doing.

4. It is esthetically unpleasing to the average medical student. He resents the mental straitjacket it forces on him, the inescapable reiteration of material he may have fully mastered. Constant turning of pages and searching for frames annoy him.

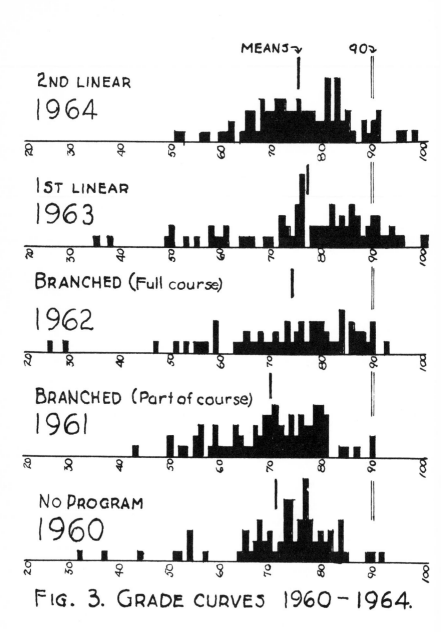

FIG. 3. GRADE CURVES 1960-1964.

We feel that our text-question design avoids these problems and also permits a desirable flexibility of approach. The student can use the program like an ordinary text by disregarding the exercises. Conversely, a sufficient expansion of the exercises can make them nearly the equivalent of a short-step program (having the advantage of the orienting textual presentation which accompanies it). And finally, the highly structured text, combined with a table of contents, provides an outline of the subject.

Although the program will not be tested on the class until next fall, we feel that we have made a major advance in separating it into two parts, a main part and a supplement. The main part contains all the concepts necessary for understanding the subject, uncluttered by qualifying details and information important only for the practice of medicine. These are provided in the supplement. The scheme offers a solution to one of the pressing problems of teaching medical students. A glance at the grade curves shows that the classes are far from homogeneous. Encouraging the slower students to largely neglect material presented to them in the supplement will, we hope, give them sufficient time to absorb the basic material and do away with the very low scores.

Our experience suggests that a program in no way suffices as a substitute for lecture, classroom discussion, or individual help. The actual effect of the program is to maintain the student in a position where he can get the optimum profit from these other activities. Printed words, in whatever form they are arranged, are cold and fixed. A subject comes alive only when it becomes associated with the human personality by means of give-and-take discussion. A concept does not become vividly real to the student until he hears it from some other person's mouth.

Coming, finally, to the matter of student reaction to the program: the heart of the problem is that the medical student has too much to do in the time available. An efficient outline is welcomed because it helps him to make short cuts. The program is less welcome because it forces him to devote full attention to each item (succeeds, in other words, in its purpose). We are hopeful that improvements in the program, particularly the segregation of secondary material into the supplement, will reduce this problem to a tolerable level.

Summary

1. A programmed presentation of the entire 100-hour course in neuroanatomy at the University of Miami School of Medicine, is reported.

2. Starting from a conventional branching program, the project has evolved over five years into a combination of structured text and student response exercises (linear form).

3. Clarity is achieved by segregating all but the basic concepts into a supplementary program. The basic concepts (some 30 to 40 per cent of the whole) are presented in an uncluttered, self-sufficient "main program." This is divided into 142 more or less homogeneous conceptual units. Each unit consists of a succinct textual presentation (average length—225 words), followed by relevant student response exercises with answers. Most units also contain review exercises designed to keep previously learned material fresh in the student's mind.

4. The most conspicuous unfavorable result has been burdening the students with increased work, resulting in decreased enjoyment of the course.

5. No controlled observations have been possible, but it appears evident that class performance has improved, as seen both in classroom activity and examinations.

6. The course has become easier to teach. Students keep pace with the lecture schedule. Many study ahead. The foundation concepts are more easily and more certainly mastered.

Programmed Instruction in Dental Anatomy*

RICHARD S. SCOTT, M.D.** and
ROBERT L. LANG, D.D.S.***

IN 1961, COOPERATIVE efforts between the University of Oregon Dental School and the Teaching Research Division of the Oregon State System of Higher Education led to a course of Programmed instruction in dental anatomy. At that time, the Teaching Research Division (then called the Teaching Research Center) was only a year old. It had been formed at the Oregon College of Education, Monmouth, Oregon, to carry out investigations of contemporary and advanced educational methods and techniques. Since then, Teaching Research has grown to full divisional status and serves all the institutions of higher learning in the state of Oregon. The division now has 45 investigators (including educational psychologists, statisticians, and media specialists) and conducts research activities in all areas of education.

Background

In September, 1961, Drs. Jack Edling and Bert Kersh (the director and associate director of Teaching Research) addressed the University of Oregon Dental School faculty on the "Principles and Practice of Programmed Learning." The subject aroused the interest of several of the dental school faculty, particularly Dr.

*Supported by the Public Health Service, U. S. Department of Health, Education and Welfare.
**Teaching Research Division, Oregon State System of Higher Education.
***University of Oregon Dental School, Portland, Oregon.

Robert L. Lang, head of the Crown and Bridge Department. Subsequent talks between Dr. Lang and the Teaching Research Division led to a proposal for a pilot project to program a segment of the dental anatomy course with the purpose of determining feasibility and effectiveness. This research was supported by the basic budget of the Teaching Research Division, by two grants from the International Research Fund of the State System, and by the University of Oregon Dental School.

Previous dental instruction

The previous course in dental anatomy had been taught using the conventional lecture method, consisting of one hour per week during the fall and winter term of the freshman year. The lectures included the use of slides showing the various teeth being studied. The lectures were supplemented by a two-hour weekly laboratory session, where construction of plaster and wax tooth models was the principal activity. The texts used were R. C. Wheeler's, *Textbook of Dental Anatomy and Physiology*[1] and *Atlas of Tooth Form.*[2]

Content of the pilot program

The program written for the pilot project involved material covered in the first four lectures of the dental anatomy course:

1) definition of terms;

2) general considerations covering the teeth and periodontal tissues;

3) arrangement of teeth (including the reference code); and

4) developmental history of the dentition.

The program contained about 500 frames altogether, using a combined linear and branching style, and was divided into four chapters. Following each chapter, an internal criterion test quizzed the student on four or five relevant subject areas developed in the chapter. Each test item had several distractors and was arranged so that missed items washed the student back into the program for remedial instruction before continuing. The program was reinforced by an eight-page overlay book that detailed many of the tooth elements studied in the course. In addition, a kit of tooth models was provided as further visual support of the program.

Administration of the pilot program

The program was given to the freshman class of 1962. It supplemented the first four lectures and the eight one-hour laboratory sessions of the first four weeks. Results showed that students completed the course in a mean time of four hours and six minutes, a 66 percent reduction over lecture-type teaching time. The fastest completion time was less than three hours; the slowest was five hours and twenty minutes. The mean score on the final examination was 89.6 percent; the mean score on a comparable test given the previous year, using conventional instruction, was 83.1 percent. Two years previously, the mean score was 83.8 percent (conventional tests and instruction). In addition, no student had ever achieved a perfect score on the conventional examination; but using the programmed material, two students received 100 percent. The program was also tried on a class of 24 dental hygienists; the mean score was 88.9 percent, against 87.1 percent scored on a comparable test following conventional instruction given the previous year. Although there were uncontrolled factors in these comparisons, the information strongly suggests that the programmed material was highly successful both in terms of efficient and effective teaching. In addition, student reception was enthusiastic.

Current efforts

With these positive results, the Teaching Research Division received a three-year grant to complete the programming of the entire dental anatomy course and to study its effectiveness. This grant, entitled *Research on Programmed Dental Instruction,* is from the Public Health Service of the U. S. Department of Health, Education and Welfare. Robert L. Lang, D.D.S., University of Oregon Dental School, is the principal investigator.

As presently outlined, the study will have five objectives:

1) To determine whether learning from programmed materials is as effective as learning from present instructional procedures;

2) to assess the acceptability of programmed self-instruction by staff and students;

3) to determine the feasibility of programmed self-instruction procedures in dental education;

4) to determine the form of programmed material best suited to selected phases of dental education; and

5) to assess the effects of an expanded curriculum in terms of additional capabilities of students.

When completed, the course will comprise four additional volumes, each comparable in size to the one in the pilot study. Volumes II and III will cover physiologic tooth form protecting the periodontium, plus detailed description of the permanent tooth groups. Volume IV will cover the deciduous dentition and the anatomy of the various root and pulp structures. Volume V will deal with occlusion and variations between teeth. All will rely extensively on captioned line art and other visual materials. In addition, the Overlay Book and Tooth Model Kit will be available for reference.

Paralleling the use of the programmed materials, the 1964-65 freshman class, serving as a control group, will also undergo conventional instruction consisting of weekly lectures and laboratory-study sessions. The resulting data will be evaluated using techniques developed by Siegel and Siegel[3]. The important considerations include consideration of scholastic aptitude, knowledge of subject matter before taking the course, motivation to learn specific content, and mind set toward education.

The instrument for measuring attitudes toward education is the I.G. Set scale, which consists of 93 items for measuring whether students are more interested in learning specific facts or principles. In addition, the subjects will report on the amount of time each student studies out of class, as well as indicating (anonymously) their reactions to the instructional sequence and instructor. To serve as dependent, or criterion, measures of performance, a specific set of behavioral objectives and tests is being developed. When this material is completed in the fall of 1965, the incoming freshman class will serve as a developmental group for the completed two-term program. After the program is given to this group, the 1966-67 class will receive the finally developed programmed texts.

Development of programmed material

The procedure followed in producing the programmed text involves the following steps: first, rough frames are written by the programmers, following a subject outline supplied by the dental school. These frames are then checked by the dental group for accuracy of subject matter, content, and terminology. Next, the frames are examined carefully to assure their following established programming techniques. Necessary visual material (line drawings, primarily) is then keyed into the text. Following this step, students (usually juniors and seniors in the sciences) read the program with a programmer to discover any areas of ambiguity or confusion in the copy or visual material. Finally the chapters are rewritten, to incorporate any changes and to introduce required new branches; they are then printed.

Summary

The pilot dental anatomy course using the programmed teaching approach has resulted in higher student test scores, reduced teaching time, and generally enthusiastic student response. Volume I of the course is now available, with Volumes II, III, IV, and V in preparation. The program will be administered during the next two years, the class of 1966-67 receiving the completed syllabus. The entire program is being prepared by the Teaching Research Division of the Oregon State System of Higher Education and the University of Oregon Dental School.

References

1. Wheeler, R. C. *A Textbook of Dental Anatomy and Physiology.* Philadelphia: Saunders, 1958.

2. Wheeler, R. C. *Atlas of Tooth Form.* Philadelphia: Saunders, 1962.

3. Siegel, L., and Siegel, L. C. "The Instructional Gestalt: A Conceptual Framework and Design for Educational Research." *Audio-Visual Communication Review.* 12:16-45 (Spring) 1964.

Progress Report on a Program of Individualized Medical Instruction

EUGENE N. GARCIA, Ph.D.* and
KENNETH H. IBSEN, Ph.D.*

AT THE FIRST Rochester Conference we reported a design for a program which provides an individualized approach to medical instruction.[1] The following is a description of our initial attempt to implement such an individualized instructional program in the biochemistry laboratory at the California College of Medicine.

The laboratory time for biochemistry was scheduled so that the students could spend one hour in study prior to beginning each experiment. After each week's laboratory work was completed, there was an additional hour for study and the discussion of both data and experiments.

The purpose of the study hour prior to the lab work was to help the students be better prepared in their approach to the lab work. Programmed material was written to provide a self-study opportunity for the students during this period. Additional programmed material was written for an hour at the end of the week to provide a follow-up on the experiments and additional information on the same topic.**

*Both Assistant Professors of Biochemistry, California College of Medicine, Los Angeles.
**Ed. Note: For related work, now at a more advanced stage of development, in a premedical laboratory course, see: Postlethwait, S. N. "Audio-Tutoring—A Practical Solution For Independent Study," *Med. & Biol. Illus.*, *XV*: 183-187, 1965.

Thirteen units were constructed, one for each of the eleven weeks in the first trimester of the course, and two for the first half of the second trimester. The first eleven chapters comprised the following topics: Acids, Bases and Buffers; Proteins and Amino Acids; Carbohydrates; Inorganic Ions and Bone; Lipids; Lipo-proteins and Steroids; Nucleic Acids; Porphyrins; Enzyme Kinetics; Isozymes; Cytochromes. The second group was devoted to experiments in Nutrition and Urinalysis; Radioisotope Counting; and the Use of C-14 in Metabolic Experiments.

This was our first programming attempt and the results were not as positive as we would have liked. We used a linear approach requiring constructed responses. The sophomore, junior, and senior medical students who had advance-tested the material for us generally liked the format, describing it as a good means for review of the subject matter.

The lab procedures were designed to illustrate biochemical principles rather than to provide the students with experience in performing clinical lab tests. Each of the students was to do the assignments individually, submitting a duplicate data sheet after each experiment so that we could follow his progress. A shortage of equipment required that some experiments be done by pairs of students, and a few by groups of four.

For the second trimester, the experiments were all designed for groups, with each individual responsible for one portion of the project. After the completion of the experiments several individuals and groups were selected to present oral reports on their findings.

The last six weeks of the lab course were devoted to individual research projects on any phase of biochemistry which the students selected. They were each assigned a faculty member whom they could consult and who would direct their research. During this period their lab time was flexible and determined by the needs of their project. At the end, each student gave an oral report.

Since this was the first year of the program, we did not plan a controlled study to compare the effectiveness of this approach to the traditional laboratory. We were here concerned with descriptive data that would suggest revisions and alterations.

We did use an extensive questionnaire to assemble student opinions and comments on this approach. Approximately 30 percent of the 96 students returned the completed questionnaire. Only two thirds of the respondents had actually read all of the programmed materials, and half believed they profited from their use. Most of the responding students pointed out that they had not received sufficient instruction in the use of the programs and only half felt that the importance of these materials had been adequately stressed.

The programmed units which the students liked most were those which had more obvious clinical implications. This same attitude was evident in the students' statements regarding the experiments which they liked most, and which were most profitable. The experiment which was most closely tied to a clinical problem was the most popular. We soon discovered that a different format for the textual material would have been more convenient. The book was arranged in four parts: I—programmed material for the introductory hours; II—data sheets for the lab experiments; III—follow-up programmed material after the lab experiments; IV—directions for the lab procedures. This bulky manual should have been divided into two separate booklets, one with programmed material, the other with the lab directions and data sheets, and it will be rearranged in this manner for the coming year.

The students also criticized the Part II experiments which they performed, but didn't successfully complete. We will eliminate this embarrassing difficulty next year by telling the students what they are intended to observe and by having them respond to the appropriate programmed material before they go into the laboratory. We have also revised the instructions to delete some flagrant errors which were introduced by the typists and which slipped by our weary-eyed proofreader.

There was no negative feeling toward the individual projects; but most of the students were indifferent. Those who did like the projects said that they had learned much from the opportunity of wrestling with problems and techniques with their own freedom to succeed or fail. This is an encouraging result, for it suggests that our eventual goal of individualized laboratory work for all students may be attainable by improvements and revisions.

Next year we plan to run a controlled experimental study testing the effectiveness of our programs against the usual lecture system. One section of the class will serve as the experimental group. They will be given the programmed material to study at the beginning of the week; the control section will attend a lecture on the same subject matter. After three weeks, the sections will be switched and the protocols continued for another three weeks. Pretests and post-tests will be given to both sections each week, so that we can get some measure of the learning rate and efficiency of our program. We plan, in addition, to extend this study into the first weeks of the second trimester.

As one consequence of the student reactions, we began developing audiovisual materials to supplement the laboratory instructions. We are using the Hughes Videosonic machine, which employs a magnetic tape for narration and automatically changes frames from a cartridge of 35 mm color slides. So far, we have completed one instructional program on the procedure for paper electrophoresis, and several other units are being constructed to cover other types of electrophoresis, chromatography, and the use of instruments to measure radioactivity. Eventually we hope to develop an array of programmed units that will allow us to forego the lecture part of the course, and permit our students to work individually with their programs under a tutorial faculty approach.

The beginnings of our work on an individualized program are far from spectacular, but a start has been made. We are in the process of learning and adjusting to our first experiences and hope in the coming year to make even faster progress toward our ultimate objectives.

References

1. Garcia, Eugene N. "A Medical Program of Individualized Instruction," in Lysaught ,J. P. (ed.) *Programmed Instruction in Medical Education,* Rochester, N. Y., The University of Rochester. 1965. pp 157-162.

Part V

Extensions of the Programming Process

Too often there has been in the public mind a preoccupation with programmed instruction as a product—rather than a recognition of it as a process. The result of this has been that people associate programs with a few, somewhat strangely, printed books, and a small number of machine gadgets. These are, however, only artifacts that accompanied a revolution in education that centered on specifying behavior, arranging learning contingencies that required this behavior, and then providing for active student interface with those contingencies. Thus, programming is a process that can take many forms, depending upon the desired goals and the students involved. Manning describes how this process can be used to produce a "programmed lecture"; Barrows reports the development of a programmed patient to aid in clinical teaching. Huber and Williamson relate how principles of programming can affect the development of films and tests, respectively, so that their instructional quality can be improved. Finally, Geis and Grubb speculate on the possibilities inherent in the wedding of computer technology with self-instructional processes.

The Programmed Lecture:
Programmed Techniques for Oral
Presentation to Large Groups

PHIL R. MANNING, M.D.*

.ONE PROBABLE REASON that the lecture has continued to be an important technique in educational circles is that it is economical of instructional time, since one teacher can perform before a large group. The standard lecture, however, suffers from the handicap that it is quite difficult for an audience to participate actively in the learning process. Listeners are relegated to a passive status. As individuals become passive, their attention may wander.

Small group teaching has the advantage of permitting considerable active participation on the part of the student. Small group teaching, however, has the disadvantage of requiring many instructors.

The concept of a programmed lecture is presented here with a view toward gaining active participation on the part of students in a large group. It is hoped that some of the advantages of small group teaching may thus be incorporated into large group sessions.

The technique itself is simple; first the lecturer decides upon the objectives of the discussion; he then formulates questions which are concerned with those objectives. For each question several optional answers are provided. The questions and answers should be short and to the point. The printed questions and answers are distributed to the audience. During the session the instructor will read the questions one by one and ask the audience to circle the correct answer.

*Associate Dean, Post-Graduate Education, University of Southern California School of Medicine.

After each member of the audience has committed himself, a discussion is carried out on various aspects of each question. Depending on the size of the group, oral participation from the audience can be encouraged or discouraged. In any event, the learner takes an active role in the lecture by committing himself on paper to one of the options. We feel that this commitment should make the learner a more active participant in the learning process of a programmed case presentation.

Example of a programmed case presentation

This 20-year-old white woman is pregnant with her first child. She was apparently totally asymptomatic until she was five months pregnant, at which time she developed a cough and running nose. There was no fever. Three days after the onset of the cold, her eyes and skin became yellow. Her skin itched, her urine was dark, and her stools were light. The signs persisted until delivery. At no time did the patient feel ill. She was not exposed to anyone with jaundice. She received no transfusions or injections. She took no medicine other than aspirin. The jaundice persisted until the time of delivery, after which it cleared.

Questions:

1. Which liver function studies do you wish to know the result of? (Circle as many as indicated)
   a. Alkaline phosphatase
   b. B.S.P.
   c. Bilirubin
   d. SGPT
   e. SGOT
   f. Urine bile
   g. Albumin globulin

After the audience commit themselves on paper, the lecturer will give the values of each test and discuss the need for the information as well as the meaning of the result of the information. The conclusion is reached that the laboratory studies indicate obstructive jaundice with no evidence of hepatocellular disease.

2. A liver biopsy was performed. What finding would you predict? (Circle one)
   a. Hepatocellular necrosis
   b. Bile stasis

    c. Granulomas
    d. Carcinoma
    e. Normal liver

Based on the liver function tests, the audience is asked to predict the microscopic picture of the liver. The instructor then indicates that bile stasis was found and reviews studies on how the liver functions.

3. What is the diagnosis? (Circle one)
    a. Infectious hepatitis
    b. Silent gallstone
    c. Benign cholestatic jaundice of pregnancy
    d. Fatty metamorphosis of the liver
    e. Carotinemia

The name of the entity under discussion is introduced and defined on the basis of liver function tests and microscopic picture.

4. Will there be any permanent disability from liver disease in the patient? (Circle one)
    a. Yes
    b. No

The point is made that the condition does not cause permanent disability.

5. May the condition be expected to recur during subsequent pregnancies? (Circle one)
    a. Yes
    b. No

The point is made that the condition may be expected to recur during subsequent pregnancies.

6. In following the patient through the pregnancy, what is the single most important laboratory test to obtain, from a practical standpoint? (Circle one)
    a. SGPT
    b. Prothrombin time
    c. Albumin globulin
    d. Urine bile
    e. Alkaline phosphatase

The practical point is made that the cholestasis might cause decreased Vitamin K absorption from the G.I. tract, with subsequent prolongation of prothrombin time and possible bleeding tendency if not corrected.

The above example was designed to meet six objectives:

1. To acquaint the audience with the entity.

2. To point out the liver function abnormalities of the condition.

3. To describe the microscopic picture of the condition.

4. To indicate that the condition is benign.

5. To indicate that the condition often recurs during subsequent pregnancies.

6. To emphasize that in this condition the prothrombin time should be followed during the pregnancy.

To date no systematic evaluation has been carried out on the effectiveness and efficiency of the programmed lecture. A detailed evaluative study is planned for the near future. However, questions have been submitted to gain the opinions of various groups that have participated in this form of teaching. Almost all members of the audiences indicated that they do, indeed, have a more active role to play in the learning process and that their attention is less likely to wander.

From the standpoint of the instructor, it would appear that it is necessary for him to be more specific in outlining his objectives, and it may be more difficult to skip over difficult or complex material. Generally speaking, the programmed lecture may take 10 to 20 percent more time to cover the material.

One might ask whether a programmed lecture has any value over a programmed text. In this regard, it can be pointed out that the preparation of a programmed lecture is a relatively simple matter, whereas a printed program is complex and time consuming. Also, in the programmed lecture there is possibility for spontaneous responses both from the instructor and from the audience. We have so far applied the approach of the programmed lecture both to case presentations (as illustrated in this paper) and to panel discussions.

The Programmed Patient: Evaluation and Instruction in Clinical Neurology

HOWARD S. BARROWS, M.D.*

EVALUATION OF STUDENTS on the neurological clinical clerkship is necessary in our view to provide a satisfactory appraisal of each student's performance, to identify the difficulties of the individual student, and to determine the effectiveness of the teaching methods used by the faculty. The goals of a clinical clerkship include helping students achieve adequate skills in history taking, physical examination, diagnosis, differential diagnosis, diagnostic procedures, and patient management. Written and oral examinations cannot adequately measure a student's performance in these areas. They can never reveal (1) how the student relates to the patient, (2) the effectiveness of his bedside manner, (3) his ability to elicit and develop an accurate history, (4) his ability to perform a correct, organized, effective physical examination, (5) his ability to identify and interpret abnormal symptoms and signs. Yet, these are skills that every recipient of an M.D. degree is expected to possess.

A clinically oriented method of testing which has been used is the direct observation of students examining patients. A serious drawback of this approach is the considerable faculty time required. In addition, the presence of an observer can alter the student-patient relationship. An alternate method is the assignment of the clinical students to patients known to the faculty. The students report their

*Associate Professor, Department of Neurology, University of Southern California School of Medicine.

findings in written or oral form. No matter how well a patient may be known by the faculty, however, there is no assurance that the patient will present the same history or even the same physical findings to the students. The patient's illness, attitudes, and memory can change from hour to hour. In addition, suitable patients are often hard to find at examination time. In this approach no information on the students' examination skills or bedside manner is obtained, and of most importance, several students generally need to be evaluated at once. If a group of students each examines a different patient, this prevents comparison among the students.

The "programmed patient" technique was devised as an attempt to develop a patient-oriented method for appraising student performance in the clinical neurological skills expected of a physician. It was designed to provide a test situation consistent from student to student and free of the variables and drawbacks mentioned above. The approach involves training a normal person in the simulation of disease. This person learns to assume and present, on student examination, a history and neurological findings in the manner of an actual patient who has existed on our service. After examination by the student, this "programmed patient" is requested to answer a questionnaire designed to determine the accuracy and completeness of the student's work-up and the "patient's" reaction to his examination and bedside technique. This also requires considerable experience and training on the part of the model simulating the patient.

During their 25 day clinical clerkship in neurology, the students are examined by the programmed patient method early enough so that information derived from this encounter may be of benefit to them. Each clerkship group consists of six or seven students. The test is performed on one morning, between 7:15 a.m. and 1 p.m. The students are scheduled to interview and examine the programmed patient as if she were a real patient. They are given a half-hour time limit. Before the student goes to examine the patient he is asked to read the following instructions:

Instructions for final test Neurology Clerkship

This person is simulating an actual neurological case seen on the ward service some time ago.

1. You are to approach, interview, and examine this person exactly as you would an actual patient, cutting no corners or avoiding any part of the examination that is indicated by the

clinical picture. We are evaluating your performance here on the assumption that you would behave identically with an actual patient.

2. Please assume the following:
   General physical examination is unremarkable except for a distended bladder on abdominal palpation.

3. You must finish in 30 minutes.

4. Write this case up as a typical ward history on No. 4 sheet.

You will note that findings on the patient are described that could not be simulated by the programmed patient. The student is to examine these, and present and use them in his evaluation. In the interest of time, we have not held the students responsible for the complete physical examination, but instead have told them what findings were present. When the student enters the room and begins his interview, the model's work begins. She carefully notes his manner, opening remarks, and general attitude. She attempts to answer questions in the manner of the patient who had the illness she is simulating. She will talk tangentially about a large number of things that are not medically valuable until the student redirects the conversation. She is completely preoccupied with her most recent or catastrophic symptoms, revealing other associated and important symptoms only to the degree with which the student interrogates. Certain symptoms, such as urinary urgency in the case for which the instructions were used, will be revealed only on direct questioning of the actual patient.

During the examination the programmed patient notes every procedure and technique the student uses, as well as the degree of gentleness and extent of organization of his approach. She notes the manner in which he uses diagnostic instruments. In the case being described here, the student finds the programmed patient to have variable sensory losses from the waist down, complete paraplegia, early spasticity in the lower extremities, bilateral Babinskis, a weak right triceps and grip, and a blind left eye. All these findings are successfully simulated by the model.

When the student is finished he is given an hour to write up the results of this history and neurological examination on the forms normally used for patients on the ward service. He is allowed to consult any textbooks or physicians in his evaluation, as would be true with an actual patient. He must, in addition, write down his diagnosis, differential diagnosis, suggested work-up, and plan of management. The students are not allowed to confer with each other during the test day (Figure 1).

The model has 10 minutes in which to complete a detailed questionnaire before the next scheduled examination by another student. The questionnaire (Figure 2) surveys all the skills and attitudes that are felt to be important in a student physician's examination of a patient.

Subsequently, a member of the faculty, using the reports from the model and the student, meets with the student, reviews the encounter, and quizzes him in depth concerning anatomy, physiology, diagnosis, and other matters related to the problem presented by the patient. In this manner the faculty member gets a very detailed idea not only of the student's intellectual capabilities, but also of his practical ability to draw conclusions from his examination of the patient. Following such a test period, the members of the faculty and the model review the experience to determine possible sources of error and possible ways to improve the next encounter.

The data produced from this technique allows the faculty to discover many problems in history taking, examination techniques, application of basic science concepts, concepts of treatment, and problems in patient rapport in the student's performance which might otherwise have gone unnoticed. The students profit by such an examination in that they receive comments and suggestions which may improve their approach and technique with patients and reveal other errors of which they were not aware. When a number of students in the clerkship are found to make common errors, the faculty has an indication of an area in which an improvement in instruction may be necessary.

The use of this approach, the programmed patient, has enabled the faculty to report much more accurately the clinical performance of students in neurology. Faculty members not privy to the information obtained through the use of a programmed-patient appraisal were unable to differentiate among six students who had just completed the 25-day clerkship in neurology. The students were all described as "somewhat above average" and "generally·unremarkable in their performance." However, using the results of the more systematic evaluation procedure, we were able to discover the outstanding

FIGURE   I

A section of the programmed patient report
form to be completed by the examining student.

OK NG
☐   ☐   APHASIA TESTING

            ☐ follow instructions
            ☐ name objects _____
            ☐ write _____
            ☐ repeat _____
            ☐ read _____
            ☐ speech _____
            ☐ other _____
                    _____

☐   ☐   SMELL _____
            ☐ together _____ ☐ nose released early _____
            ☐ eyes open _____ ☐ scent used _____

☐   ☐   VISUAL ACUITY _____
            ☐ together _____
                                              ☐ object _____

☐   ☐   VISUAL FIELDS _____
            ☐ together _____
                                              not in four directions _____

☐   ☐   OPHTHALMOSCOPE _____
            ☐ not dark _____
            ☐ vision obscured _____ ☐ directions unclear _____
                                                ☐ other _____

☐   ☐   PUPILLARY REACTION TO LIGHT _____

☐   ☐   PUPILLARY REACTION TO NEAR VISION _____

student of the six as well as one who was clearly deficient. Furthermore, the students' specific performance characteristics—particularly
those which established the difference between the outstanding student and the others and between the deficient student and the rest—
were objectively identified, systematically recorded, and appropri-
ately reported. Students judged by this procedure, furthermore, re-
acted favorably and expressed satisfaction with having been
"graded" in such a realistic and objective manner. They found the
testing situation stimulating and fair.

FIGURE   2

A section of the programmed patient report form to be completed by the "patient" following the examination.

EXAMINER'S ATTITUDE:

☐ COMPETENT _____
☐ INSECURE _____
☐ PUZZLED _____
☐ HESITANT _____
☐ PLEASANT _____
☐ REASSURING _____
☐ COLD _____
☐ BRUSQUE _____
☐ TOO FUNNY _____
☐ TOO SERIOUS _____
☐ OTHER _____

EXAMINER'S APPROACH:

☐ INTERESTED _____
☐ COURTEOUS _____
☐ NO OPENER _____
☐ NO INTRODUCTION _____
☐ OTHER _____

EXAMINER'S MANNER:

☐ ROUGH _____
☐ GENTLE _____
☐ FEARFUL _____
☐ REASSURING _____
☐ OTHER _____

Instructional application

In a modified manner, the programmed patient has also been used as a subject for post-graduate workshops in settings where patients were impossible to obtain, such as hotels, resort areas, and small towns. One well-trained model, during a workshop in Hawaii, was able to simulate 15 different patients. In this procedure, the instruc-

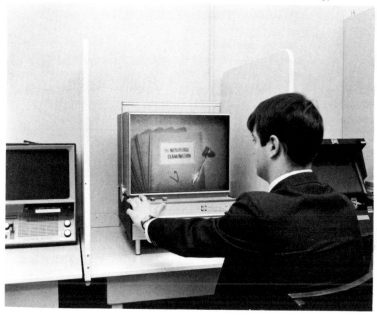

FIGURE 3 - Student using a self-instructional film on neurology developed out of the "programmed patient" project.

tor in the workshop reads a brief history selected from departmental files because of its instructive value. The model lies before the group gowned and on a makeshift table, arranged as a bed, in the manner of a patient. The physicians in the group are asked what additional information concerning the patient they want. This is provided from the actual record. A volunteer is asked to examine the patient, concentrating on the areas pertinent to the problem identified in the history. In a workshop atmosphere this is done with suggestions from the group and guidance by the instructor on technique, interpretation, etc. In this encounter the model need not memorize the details of the history but only simulate the abnormal findings, thus allowing her a greater repertoire. Subsequently, volunteers in the group are asked to describe their diagnoses, differential diagnoses, work-up procedure, plan of management, etc. In such a protocol any didactic information previously planned can be elaborated in the structure of the clinical presentation.

This technique in the post-graduate workshop encourages interest and participation by the physicians and keeps the discussion centered on the problem of a living human. While the model is admittedly a counterfeit patient, she more strongly resembles a patient with the clinical problem than do slides, movies, or syllabi. There is a distinct advantage over a real patient in that examination and discussion of all aspects of neurological illness can be done in the presence of this simulated patient. The presentation of the history by the instructor not only saves time in this workshop situation but obviates the need for the model to spend extensive preparation time in learning the history. Her efforts are limited to learning the simulation of signs.

Conclusion

The programmed patient provides a well-controlled but *clinical* test of student performance that measures bedside manner, examination technique, and clinical ability, all of which are essential to the good physician. Despite its "gimmicky" quality, students and faculty have been enthusiastic with its results. In the postgraduate workshop the programmed patient has kept the meetings patient oriented, despite exotic or holiday surroundings in areas where patients are impossible to obtain.

I wish to make it absolutely clear that this technique is not intended as a substitute for patients, whom our students work with in abundance. It is offered, rather, as an adjunct to neurological teaching.

The development and application of this technique has been formulated in conjunction with Dr. Stephen Abrahamson, Director of our Division of Research in Medical Education.

Programmed Motion Picture Films

JOHN FRANKLIN HUBER, M.D.*

As AN EDUCATOR I have, of course, been interested in the potentials of programmed learning. As an anatomist I have been interested in what appear to me to be special problems related to the programming of learning in anatomy.

In considering the use of programmed learning in anatomy, the fact that the learning and understanding of structure can best be accomplished by visual means leads to the belief that the usual type of verbal programming is not an ideal learning approach for the subject matter of anatomy. If this premise can be accepted, consideration might first be given to a lavish use of illustration combined with verbal programming in which the word content is keyed to the printed visual material in a programmed book. Such an approach would require an extensive use of excellent illustrations which would be expensive and which, unless the pictures were in three-dimension with a proper viewer, would lack something in the way of the impression of depth that is so desirable.

Another possible approach to programmed learning in anatomy could be the use of a specially designed teaching machine which would allow one to view stereo pairs such as the ones in Dr. David Bassett's excellent stereo *Atlas of Anatomy* (published in the View-Master format) with perhaps the successive addition of labels to the pictures as step by step description and questioning is progressing in the machine. A machine with this potential, although possible, would be somewhat difficult to develop and undoubtedly rather expensive.

*Temple University School of Medicine.

Still another possibility in the programming of anatomical knowledge is one of some compromise, but one which can be readily worked out with "hardware," some of which has already been developed and more of which is in the process of development. The hardware to which I am referring is the cartridge-loading 8 mm motion picture equipment which is so well adapted to the self-instructional approach. With such equipment, it is possible to present considerations of structure in a way that makes use of many of the important principles of programmed learning and presents structure in a visual fashion with verbal reinforcement and with a definite amount of depth perception (the planned slow movement of models and specimens in the motion picture gives the viewer an impression of depth).

An experimental "programmed" motion picture of the variety described above has been produced at the Audiovisual Facility of the United States Public Health Service with my participation. This film is considered an experiment, but also a possible prototype of films which might be extremely useful in the learning of anatomy. This could be especially true if the subject matter of the films were carefully chosen and were material which students ordinarily find difficult to understand.

In order to give you a much better concept of this experimental, programmed, self-instructional film it will be shown to you in the 16 mm form from which the 8 mm copies have been made.

(*Showing of a few minutes of the "programmed" film—"Mechanisms of the Intrinsic Muscles of the Larynx."*)

The purpose of this film is to give the student an opportunity not only to learn the names of basic structures involved and to visualize their positions and relationships, but also to understand rather than learn by rote memory the mechanics involved in the changes in the larynx necessary for speech and respiration.

The principles used in constructing the film were:

1. Logical arrangement of material covered, so that each added bit of information is laid upon a foundation of the material which has already been made part of the individual's knowledge.

2. Increments of knowledge small enough that they can be readily and rapidly comprehended in light of what has already been learned.

3. Anatomy can best be learned and remembered by visual memory, which is the means of this presentation—landmarks pointed to and named instead of word descriptions.

4. Questions which are interposed are introduced as review exercises, but it is important that the review is done in the form of questions rather than repeated presentation, because the student is thus involved actively rather than passively.

5. At the end of the time interval allowed for the student to think or perhaps preferably write his answer, the correct answer to the question is given and acts as reinforcement for the student.

Such a film does not, of course, allow the student to progress at his own rate, which is one of the principles of programmed learning, but this is part of the compromise referred to earlier. It seems probable that an estimated average time for response can turn out to be satisfactory in a *relatively* homogeneous group of students such as a medical school class. If the time factor should be considered extremely important, the possibility of stopping the projector can be built into the system. On the other hand, the person who learns slowly can repeat the viewing of the film very readily in the self-instructional situation.

A version of the experimental film on the larynx without the interposed questions is being put together. This will make it possible to structure experimental studies on the value of the questions in initial learning and in retention of material learned.

The ways in which such films can be used are multiple. Some of these will be mentioned, but no attempt will be made to mention all the possible uses of films of this type.

It is possible to use such a film in the 16 mm form as part of a large group presentation on the general subject matter, a portion of which is presented in the film. The film can then be available to students after such a presentation in the cartridge-loading 8 mm format to look at again for review and mastering of whatever details are of interest.

Such a programmed film can be available in a self-instructional situation (in the library or a special self-instructional area in a department) as a primary source of knowledge which might or might not be an assigned topic for a small group discussion. The viewing of the film at his own time and as many times as he wishes might be the student's only exposure to the particular subject matter covered by the film.

I would like to suggest that it would be possible to work out a series of 8 mm cartridge-loaded films (either with or without questions included as may seem preferable after further experimentation on this point) which could present the basic science information that is part of a residency program in any medical specialty. If this were done, and the library of films and a projector were available in the specialty department, the resident could at any free time review on a self-instructional basis the basic science subject matter pertinent to his studies. Such an arrangement might be especially good for a residency program in a community hospital, but could also work well even in a university situation where it might be very difficult to schedule basic science instruction in relation to the service activities of the resident.

Programmed Tests in Assessing Clinical Judgment

JOHN W. WILLIAMSON, M.D.*

ON A WARM afternoon in Averagetown, U.S.A., Mrs. I. M. Concerned, a 38-year-old mother of three children, is seated in front of Dr. Jones' desk and nervously exclaims: "Doctor, on a recent insurance exam, I was told that I have very high blood pressure and should see you right away. Do you think it is serious?" At that moment, Dr. Jones will make the first of a series of decisions that will have profound significance in determining the future course of this patient's life. Unknown to him is the fact that Mrs. Concerned will soon develop malignant hypertension due to unilateral renal artery disease.

Although Dr. Jones wants very much to provide this patient with care that is as effective and as efficient as possible, there is increasing evidence that he will probably fall far short of this goal. As a result, the patient will likely suffer needless disability and possibly premature death because of deficiencies in this doctor's clinical judgment.

In the medical profession today there is serious need for more practical measures of the ability to solve problems, both for education and accreditation. Recently, technics of programmed testing have been developed that may provide a means of filling this need.

*Research Associate, Office of Research in Medical Education, University of Illinois College of Medicine.

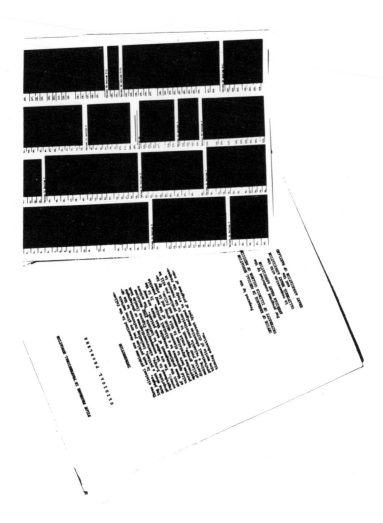

Figure 1

Patient Management Problem Booklet

and Answer Sheet

Two methods are currently being explored; both are outgrowths of the "tab test" technic developed to assess diagnostic ability of Air Force maintenance personnel.[1] The first, a linear type, was introduced to medicine by the National Board of Medical Examiners,[2] and by Rimouldi.[3] The second, a branched type, was developed by Christine McGuire and her associates at the University of Illinois.[4,5,6] This paper will describe the branched type of programmed test, and briefly outline our experience with this instrument.

The patient management problem

Essentially, a "Patient management problem" consists of a test booklet and an answer sheet for recording responses (figure 1). The test booklet presents a clinical problem together with a long list of possible diagnostic and therapeutic interventions (figure 2). The examinee is instructed to read the introductory description of the problem and then to select only those procedures which he feels are indicated in this situation. He makes each selection by erasing the overlay of the item on the answer sheet which corresponds to the request, procedure or judgment he has made. Erasing the overlay reveals information which provides either diagnostic data or the patient's response to the selected therapeutic approach. He uses the newly acquired information in making subsequent decisions about further management. For example, a problem might read:

Patient IC

Mrs. IC is a new patient who was referred to you with a history of shortness of breath and recent visual difficulties. She is obese and exhibits rather labored respiration.

In your approach to this patient you would first:
(Choose only one)

1. Obtain a brief history
2. Perform a physical examination
3. Order laboratory studies
4. Start therapy

If the physician selects Item 2 (physical examination), his erasure of that item on the answer sheet would direct him to the section with the options shown in figure 3. Suppose the physician now wishes to check vital signs (Item 11 in the list of procedures). He turns to the answer sheet, erases the overlay for Item 11 and reads "BP 138/90; P 116; R 32 per minute; T 98.6." Suppose he then elects to examine

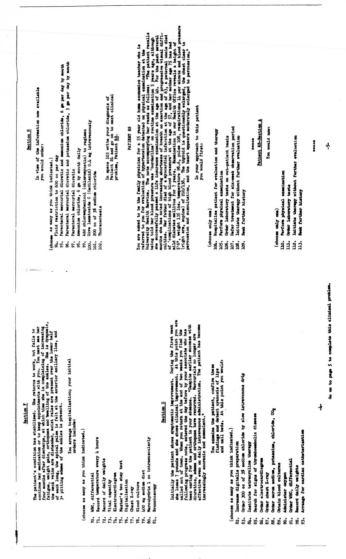

Figure 2

Simulated Patient Problem

item layout in test booklet

the heart. On erasing Item 15, he reads: "Point of maximum impulse 3cm. lateral to midclavicular line; heart tones obscured by presence of rales." If he requests X-rays, ECGs, or visible physical findings such as eye grounds, he is provided with high-quality photographs for his analysis. In this manner, the physician is called upon to make clinical decisions which simulate those he would make in practice. The answer sheet, while providing feedback to the doctor, also yields an objective record of his course of management.

Once his decisions have been made and recorded, the physician's performance may be compared with accepted criteria to establish a judgment of quality. Criteria are developed by specialists, who classify each item on a scale ranging from "very helpful" to "very harmful." Items are used only if there is definite agreement on classification. Implicit in such an instrument is the further requirement that all procedures (items) classified as "helpful" also be considered *necessary*.

Judgments of competence are made by checking the physician's selections against the prior classifications to establish two basic scores: an Efficiency Index (EI), defined as the percentage of the physician's total selections which were helpful; and a Proficiency Index (PI), inferred from the extent of agreement with the criterion group in both selecting beneficial and avoiding harmful interventions. Using these indices, performance can be analyzed for individuals or groups (such as hospital staffs or practice specialties); for diseases (such as congestive failure or hypertension) or disease combinations (cardiovascular disease, for example); or for functional categories (such as history or physical examination).

Physician performance with programmed tests

On the basis of results we have obtained for 141 volunteer practitioners, including generalists and specialists, from widely separated geographic areas, we can predict that on our illustrative branched programmed patient management test, the following will apply to the typical physician:

1) His chances of making a definitive diagnosis are slightly better than 1 in 3.

2) He probably will not obtain two thirds of the diagnostic information experts consider essential.

3) The chance that he will provide this patient definitive

PHYSICAL EXAMINATION

(Choose as many as you think indicated.)

11. CHECK VITAL SIGNS
12. EXAMINE NECK
13. EXAMINE CHEST
14. DO A COMPLETE NEUROLOGICAL EXAM
15. EXAMINE THE HEART
16. DILATE PUPILS FOR FUNDOSCOPIC EXAM
17. EXAMINE FOR ADENOPATHY

Figure 3

Simulated Patient Problem – illustrative items and answer sheet feedback treatment, which in this case might be necessary to save her life, is less than 1 in 3.

4) Of the therapeutic decisions he *will* make, 2 out of 5 will be harmful and 1 out of 5 very harmful, according to expert judgment.

Cardiologists assembled by the American Heart Association in three sections of this country, including faculty members from several major universities, examined these programmed test results and expressed the opinion that these findings are compatible with their personal experience with the usual physician management of this disease.

Evidence accumulated from other such tests reveals similar discrepancies between the clinical judgment of practicing physicians and that of recognized experts in an alarming proportion of disease areas checked thus far. Since many of these findings have been supported by recent observational studies of medical practice,[7,8] it would seem rather urgent that these discrepancies be further explored. If the results of such programmed tests prove valid, the use of this instrument for educational diagnostic purposes could have important implications in facilitating improved quality of patient care.

Summary

The need for a practical means of assessing clinical judgment would seem critical in the education and accreditation of physicians. The programmed test may offer a promising means of filling this need. This paper has described the branched form of this instrument, together with a few illustrative results of such tests administered to practicing physicians.

References

1. Glaser, Robert, *et al.* "The Tab Item: A Technic for Measurement of Proficiency in Diagnostic Problem Solving Tasks," *Education and Psychological Measurements,* Vol 14, No. 2, 1954. (Reprinted in *Teaching Machines and Programmed Learning—a Source Book*, Lumsdaine and Glaser (ed.), National Education Association of the United States, 1960.)

2. Hubbard, J. P. *Programmed Testing in Examinations and their role in evaluation of medical education and qualification for practice.* Philadelphia: National Board of Examiners, 1964, pp. 102-114.

3. Rimoldi, H. J. A. "Rationale and Application of the Test of Diagnostic Skills." *Journal of Medical Education.* 38:364-373, 1963.

4. McGuire, Christine and Babbott, David. "Simulation Technic in the Measurement of Problem Solving Skills: A Technological or Conceptual Breakthrough." Paper read at American Educational Research Association meeting, Chicago, 1965.

5. Williamson, John. "Assessing Clinical Judgment." *Journal of Medical Education.* 40:180-187, Feb., 1965.

6. Lewy, A. "Reliability of Patient Management Problems." Paper read at Colloquium on Research in Medical Education, Chicago, Dec., 1964.

7. Peterson, O. L., Andrews, L. P., Spain, R. S. and Greenberg, B. G. "An Analytical Study of North Carolina General Practice 1953-1954." *Journal of Medical Education,* 31: Part 2, December, 1956.

8. Clute, K. F. *The General Practitioner.* Toronto, Canada: The University of Toronto Press, 1963.

Computer-Assisted Instruction: Current Applications

GEORGE L. GEIS*

MY COLLEAGUE at the Center, Karl Zinn, tells this story. A man who was operated upon for a hand injury asked his doctor, "Will I be able to play the piano?" The doctor replied, "Yes, you will be able to." The patient smiled and said, "That's good. I've never been able to play it before."

The computer does not represent a magical instrument which will allow the teacher to "play the piano" when he never knew how to play it previously. Certainly with all our complaints about hardware limitation, the most inflexible component of the system is usually the instructor or the generator of computer-based materials. All of the constraints that apply to programmed instruction apply to that particular instance of programmed instruction called computer-based instruction. Thus, one cannot escape the necessity of stating objectives or of student testing by working with a machine instead of a student or an editor.

As I look at the computer, from the point of view of a non-computer man, it can possibly provide several advantages. At our Center we are interested in the behavior of authors of instructional material as much as we are interested in the behavior of students exposed to that material. We look upon the computer as a possible *author "shaper."* For several reasons we think the computer might develop,

*Center for Research on Learning and Teaching, The University of Michigan.

in the author, behaviors that are hard for us to develop in face-to-face instruction. For example, he must learn to talk to the computer. I don't simply mean learning a computer language, such as Coursewriter. I mean, instead, that he must make his instructional goals explicit, he must specify those answers he will accept, and so forth. Sometimes it is hard to insist upon this if one is working with an author, but the computer is patient and rigid about such requirements. A related advantage is that the computer can feed back to him rather soon after gathering it, data both in raw and summary form. This, as you know, is a difficult thing to do when instructional material is being tested by other means. Thirdly, the computer allows easy revision. Once materials are produced and printed, chances of extensive revision taking place are dramatically reduced. While the material remains on the computer, changes can be made simply, and probably are more likely to be made.

Still another advantage of the computer seems to be that *complex presentations* are possible using the device. This would apply not only to multimedia inputs to the student, but also to complex sequencing and instructional strategies which the computer makes possible. While I am always suspicious that an author may become bogged down in the format, especially when it is as glamorous as a computer-controlled multimedia input, the computer offers a convenient way to contrast various sequences or various means of presentation. I think it will serve a valuable purpose.

The *comparator function* of the computer is an exciting advantage. I have mentioned before that the computer must know what answers are acceptable, and therefore the author may be pressured to spell out classes of acceptable behaviors much more clearly than he ordinarily would. The comparator function also means that we can self-instruct in situations in which the student is not able to discriminate whether he is correct or not (for example, in teaching second-language pronunciation).

Complex skills, again thinking of second-language learning as an example, can be developed by the computer. The computer has two major assets in comparison with a living instructor. It has the previously mentioned discriminative ability, the comparator function. This may well be better than the discriminative ability of the instructor. The SAID system at the Center for Research on Language Behavior at the University of Michigan* can make discriminations

*See, Buiten, R. and Lane, H. L. A self-instructional device for conditioning accurate prosody. IRAL, Vol. 3, No. 3, 1965, pp. 205-219.

in vocal pitch, intensity and duration that are beyond the discriminative ability of even the best trained language teacher. The computer not only has a keen ear or eye but also is endlessly patient. The slow shaping of complex skills, then, seems a natural area for computer use, although it has been a neglected area with few exceptions up until now.

The *adaptive* capacity of an instructional system can, in theory at least, be vastly increased by using the computer. Adjustments in the path the student is following can readily be made—adjustments on the basis of previous student response. Thus, the instructional sequence can be tailored to the student. The computer in its managerial role can vary the mode of instruction as well, providing at the moment what the diagnostician has previously decided would be the best "media mix" for a student exhibiting a given performance. That record-keeping easily gets out of hand, any teacher can aver. No matter how concerned he is in adjusting to a given student, the teacher simply does not have at hand, or cannot quickly scan and digest, the complete relevant past history of the student. Computer experts tell me this is certainly feasible behavior for the machine. If so, I am excited not about the computer managing a three-ring circus of audiovisual aids (though I appreciate that ringmaster role), but about the "intelligent" managing of entry points, branching, sequencing, etc., for instruction, dynamically adjusting instruction to the past history and the immediate past behavior of each student.

For these reasons, I think, I am excited about the possible use of a computer in education in general. Now I would like to add one use that is rarely thought of in professional education. Doctors now being trained in medical school will undoubtedly use the computer as an important part of their professional equipment. We already are working on systems of information retrieval for the health sciences which would not be possible without the computer. The day is not far off when the physician will be able to dial for a specific journal article, drug information, and the like. I expect that not much further away is the time when a computer may be an important adjunct to diagnosis. I would suggest, then, that the medical student should be taught about the computer even if he is not being taught by the computer.

We will reserve for the later discussion section, such problems as:

what are the appropriate conditions for using computer-based instruction? What are some of the problems to be faced when using a computer-based instructional system, (e.g., expense)? And I hope we will have a chance to discuss the underlying bias of most people in computer-based instruction in regard to the role of error in learning and teaching.

Computer Assisted Instruction—
The Technology

RALPH E. GRUBB, Ph.D.*

AFTER APPROXIMATELY a decade of programmed instruction, it is tempting to stand back for a moment and take an inventory of where we stand. What implications have developed? What have been the broad trends? Where are we going?

I find that a number of people have reached the conclusion that programmed instruction, as we traditionally define it, has been characterized by a negatively accelerated growth curve for some time. Perhaps the chief reason for this is the *limited technology* with which it was identified. There is only so much one can do, for example, with some elementary pre-wired logic in front of the student. This is true whether it be a programmed text or a black box we call a teaching machine.

By and large, I would suggest the promises made a few years ago that programmed instruction would break the lock step of education have resulted in little more than the lock stepping of students through linear programs. It seems ironic that so many of the psychologists involved in developing such programs have overlooked the very topic that caused scientific psychology to come into existence— individual differences.

Scrambled texts and multiple choice teaching machines, of course, attempted to break out of this pattern. However, a fair amount of

---

*Educational Psychologist, Data Processing Division of the IBM Corporation, and Research Associate, Columbia University.

suspicion still persists that these alternatives merely teach the student improved error discrimination rather than providing him with increased course facility.

My previous observation concerning the relevance of technology to these learning issues may create the impression that I believe education is primarily a hardware problem. Quite the contrary. Education is, and continues to be, a software problem. The point at issue is whether the technology is adequate to carry out the instructional requirements defined by the educator, requirements which increasingly include: *simulation; computing; editing;* and *record keeping.*

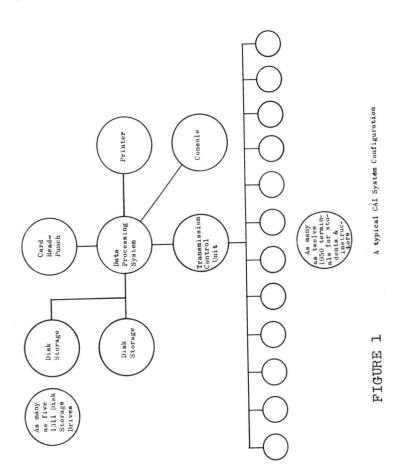

FIGURE 1   A typical CAI System Configuration

It would be difficult, if not impossible, for instructional devices of lesser logic than a computer to carry on all these activities. Since the computer is capable of simulating devices of lesser logic than itself, however, it enables comparison studies to be made, within the same medium, on several alternatives to each of these instructional requirements.

Because of this fundamental capability, a number of investigators began to explore the area of Computer-Assisted Instruction (CAI) as part of an ongoing program of research and development at the Thomas J. Watson Research Center. Our two objectives were: to configurate the technology and appropriate software needed to carry out the educational activities mentioned; and to investigate subsequent teaching/learning techniques.

Hardware

Our presently constituted CAI system includes: a central processing system, such as a 1401, 1440, or 1460; a transmission control unit; disk storage units; and student/author typing stations.

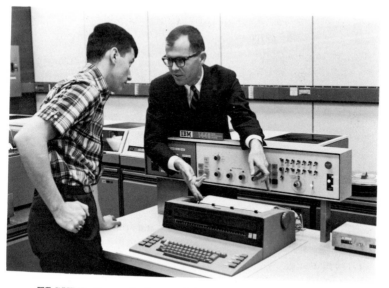

FIGURE 2 - I B M 1440 data processing system with 1311 disk storage units in background.

The central processor is the intermediary between the students and the course material in the disk storage. Curriculum sequences written by the author are placed into disk storage and retrieved by the processor for presentation to the student/teaching stations. A further function for the central processing unit is to process students' answers and to assemble courses.

Computerized typewriters serve as the interface between the students and/or authors and the central processing unit. Because this is a data communications system, ordinary voice-grade telephone lines serve as the link between the terminals and the transmission control unit.

Because the system works so rapidly, the individual is not aware that the system is also working for other students and/or authors at the same time. The present system handles 12 typewriter terminals, more or less simultaneously.

Software

It became apparent at the start of the project that the bottleneck in CAI lay in course development. One of the particular reasons for this in our system was the requirement that any author be schooled in complicated computer programming languages, or have ready assistance available from someone possessing this knowledge.

A better solution to this problem was found by developing a simple interpretive author entry language called COURSEWRITER. Through observation and analysis, we discovered that approximately one dozen operation codes could handle the majority of conditions found in current simulated tutorial dialogues. Special instances in response processing could be handled by calling for subroutines written in the machine language, thereby making COURSEWRITER an open-ended language.

By using simple two-letter operation codes in COURSEWRITER, the author merely tags each statement in his program with one of these codes to indicate its desired effect on the student. He does not have to concern himself personally with the computer's organization of the material. Thus, in a simplified manner the author builds in any logical flow of material that is consistent with his teaching philosophy. Moreover, the executive routine in the central processor permits authors to work simultaneously with students, with the instructors typing in their educational programs remotely from any of the communicating typing stations.

Registers are also available in COURSEWRITER and can be used as n-counters if the author chooses. By adding weighted values to the various registers as a function of the student's performance, the author can keep detailed records on the response history of each student. The author can use these data in the course itself by having the control program continually interrogate the contents of the n-counters. If the content of a particular counter is greater than or equal to a specified value, the program can automatically branch to some appropriate place in the course. Thus, the author is able to dynamically adjust the presentation of course material as a function of the student's response history.

Ten control words also permit the author to revise his course material at any point. Since the students are sharing this particular course in the computer's memory, this means that real time changes immediately update the course for everyone. This is in sharp contrast to the usual procedure for field testing less sophisticated learning programs. There you must recall experimental copies and produce revised editions which are both costly and time-consuming.

Instructional material may be presented orally or visually in a CAI medium. A special audiovisual device connected to the typing

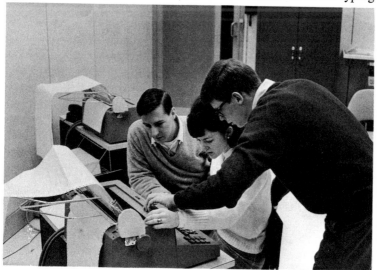

FIGURE 3 - Students and I B M 1050 data communications terminals.

station is under control of the course logic. Thus, the author can display taped sequences or slides correlated with the instructional program, all in the COURSEWRITER language.

Teaching techniques

The following sequences of interaction between the student and the computer illustrate the conversational interaction possible in the CAI medium.

1) Statistics

The first is a sample from one of the earliest courses, a psychological statistics course.

It will be seen that, when the student signed on for this particular day, the computer automatically picked him up from his previous work.

We see that he was given a reading assignment in a loose-leaf text, and then questioned on the material. His first answer was in-

J. A. Tirrell stat-001

READ SECTIONS 8. 7 - 8. 13
9. The standard error of the difference is a _____ _____
computed on mean differences rather than sample means.

difference score

How can the standard error of the difference be a difference score when it is really a measure of variability? Try again.

standard deviation

10. The symbol for the standard error of the difference is
_____ .

s_d

Lower case "s" please. Type correct answer.

s_d

11. Compute the s_d for two large samples whose

$s_{\overline{x}_1} = .75$ and $s_{\overline{x}_2} = .69.$

Figure 4. Sample typeout from student in psychological course.

correct, so the computer issued an appropriate hint based on his response. The author here has used a guided discovery technique in a conversational mode to lead the student to his own insightful solution. The computer is following the author's commands to give the student a graded prompt. Following the author's instruction it can even break the material down into remedial sequences.

In an earlier version of this course the student did all his computing through the same computer facility. This was accomplished by a "super desk calculator" routine on disk storage which treated the student's typewriter as a simulated desk calculator when requested.

2) German

In this instance, we see a student's efforts on a German translation exercise written by scientists at the Thomas J. Watson Research Center. This particular lesson incorporates a dictionary look-up feature which the computer supplies.

The student asked for a translation of the words "house," "ask," and "for," by using the slash as a delineating character. The computer responded with the appropriate translation as requested and then the student attempted the answer. The author may call in subroutines to operate on the student's answer if no exact match occurs between the input response and the target answer.

```
09/02/65  13:12
J. A. Tirrell  gerdic 1

When you come to the house, ask for Mr. Tailor.

/
house ask for
/

        das Haus = house
        fragen = to ask
        nach = for

Wenn Sie ins Haus kommt, fragen sie nack Herrn Schneider.

    Wenn Sie --- Haus komm --, fragen _ ie nach Herrn Schneider.
```

Fig. 5. Sample typeout from student in a German dictation exercise.

Subroutines already developed will look for key words that the author specifies, or compare strings of characters with the target answer, as in the above figure. The author specified in this instance that the computer give back to the student those parts of his answer which were correct, as shown on the last line of the figure. This selective feedback permits the student to concentrate on erroneous parts of his answer and correct them.

Since the author can specify the limits within which a student response can vary and still be considered correct by the computer in its "editing routines," it can be a dynamic variable manipulated from question to question.

3) Bridge

An increasingly important activity in an educational setting is that of simulation. While computers have transacted decision games with players for many years, these have largely been an adjunct to instructional courses and the players frequently have waited hours or days for the results of their decision making. What are the educational possibilities if this process were done in "real" time and inextricably bound to the ongoing course material?

An illustration that may be emblematic of such an approach is the following CAI demonstration sequence from a hand of bridge. Written at the Thomas J. Watson Research Center, it demonstrates the effects of programming a truncated tree structure of contingencies in the COURSEWRITER language.

```
1s
        W-p N-2h E-4c
        OK.  It's your bid again.
4s
        W-p N-p E-5c
        Well, what do you say over five clubs?
P
        W-p N-5s E-p
        Your bid.
P
        West leads the diamond king.  What do you play?
d-4
        E-d2
d3
        Their trick.
        W-c8
```

cj

E-ck

c4

Their trick.
E-ca

s2

W-c7 N-cq
Your lead.

s10

W-s6
And from the dummy?

s7

E-s3
Next?

sk

Input error? Try again.

sk

Input error? Try again.

sa

Input error? Try again.

s4

W-s8 N-sk E-c2
Next?

h6

E-h3, S-hk, W-h2
Next?

ha

W-h4, N-h7, E-c3
Next?

s5

W-s9, N-sa, E-c6
Next?

hq

E-c9, S-d6, W-h5
Next?

h8

Please repeat

h8

E-d5
And from your hand?

sj

W-hj

You still must lose a diamond for down 1.
You can make 5 spades. Would you like to
try again? (yes or no)

Yes

Before another try let's consider the situation
further. If at any point in this sequence you are
sure that you see how to play the hand you may
bypass the remainder and replay the hand by
entering "ok". After you gain the lead you
must take all eleven tricks. How many trump
tricks can you take?

6

Right. How many club tricks can you take?

0

Right, you can't take any tricks in clubs.
How many diamond tricks can you take without
first giving up the lead?

FIGURE 6 - Sample typeout from
student in the bridge game.

The computer starts the dialogue by typing "Study your hand.
You are dealer, so bid when you are ready." After the player (South)
typed 1s (for one spade), it quickly bid for his opponents and his
partner: W-p, N-2h, E-4c. That, of course, was simply shorthand
notation for saying the West passed, North bid two hearts and East
responded with four clubs.

The implications of such a gaming sequence for instruction in
areas like medical diagnosis and laboratory skills are, of course,
obvious.

Research studies

It would be presumptuous to label this section as "results" since
our early studies are more suggestive than conclusive. One of the
early pilot studies, done with a special terminal connected to the
IBM 650 computer, studied the effects of computer tutoring of steno-
typing. Dr Uttal[5] discovered in that project that with only 50 hours
of instruction at the computer terminal, college students were performing at a level equivalent to that of persons exposed to as much
as 200-300 hours of conventional instruction. A pilot study[1] designed to explore the teaching of statistics, evidenced an equally
dramatic time savings coupled with a high level of terminal performance.

A more recent study[2] with the same statistics course has produced several findings with wide implication for further research in CAI. We attempted to study the effects of paired student interaction at the computer terminals. Thirty college students were selected for this experiment on a predictor variable, CEEB scores (verbal only), resulting in a 2 x 2 factorial design whose elements were: high pairs; low pairs; high controls; and low controls. The controls worked alone in contrast to their paired associates.

Analysis of variance indicated that: (1) there was no difference in final performance on an individually written examination among and between the four treatment groups; and (2) pairs of students completed the course as quickly as did the controls. Questionnaire results indicated that many of the students preferred the pairing arrangement and favored working with a partner.

If these results can be found by experimenters employing other subject matters and predictor variables, there will be increased hope for social interaction within the teaching conditions of CAI for small groups. Certainly, there are obvious economic advantages, since one can reduce the cost of the educational terminal device by a factor of two in the process.

A study comparing the effects of three modes of instruction in FORTRAN was undertaken by Dr. Schurdak.[4] The treatment groups consisted of: (1) CAI (C); (2) programmed text (P); and (3) text with workbook exercises (T). Sixteen college students served in each of the 3 conditions resulting in a total of 48 students. Figure 7 summarizes the performance of the three experimental groups on the criterion test. The abscissa is the Henmon-Nelson total score for the students.

An analysis of covariance disclosed that the differences among the means of the three treatments were significant, $F = 6.50$, df 2, 44, $p < .01$. While group C was significantly higher than P, the difference between P and T was not significant. Using as covariates either of the two separate types of scores given by the Henmon-Nelson Test, verbal and quantitative, the results were essentially the same.

It can be seen in figure 7 that students with high Henmon-Nelson scores appear to obtain approximately the same scores on the criterion test in each experimental treatment, i.e., the regression lines appear to converge for high Henmon-Nelson scores. Conversely,

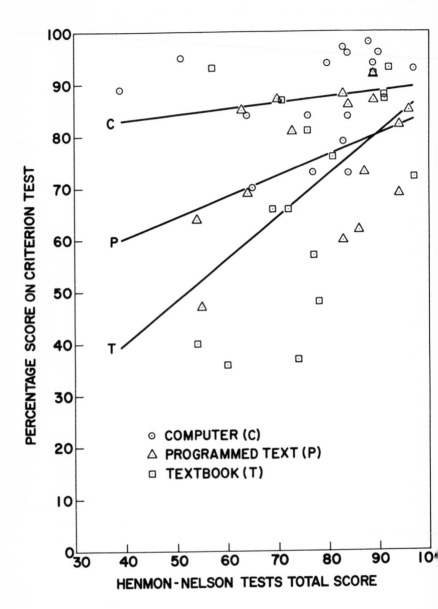

Figure 7. Regression of criterion test score on total Henmon–Nelson score for computer (C), programmed text (P), and textbook (T) groups.

students with lower Henmon-Nelson scores perform quite differently on the criterion tests in the three treatment groups. Thus, individualized instruction seems to offer real advantage to lower ability students without acting as an impediment to the high ability learners.

Discussion

These preliminary studies seem to indicate that the computer offers substantial advantages to the instructional process. How widely these observations can be generalized is, of course, a question for continuing research.

The extent to which CAI can free the educator for more creative interactions with his students is, in and of itself, a matter of great value. Public education, alone, suffers from a shortage of approximately 250,000 teachers this year; other portions of the academic institution face similar difficulties. One solution to a teacher shortage is to make the most efficient use possible of our present faculties. CAI offers some unique possibilities for the improvement of educational research. Perhaps for the first time in the history of education we are able to capture a wealth of meaningful student data as it is created in on-going course sequences. The use of "real time" clock in a computer system, for example, enables us to measure the latency for each individual item in an instructional course. Since we find in many instances a high positive correlation between increased item latency and student tendency to err, immediate revision can be considered (for example, anticipatory cueing might be invoked) on the basis of early users' experience, so that later users will find their path smoothed.

Another possibility concerns the use of psychological tests in a CAI medium. By simply entering a standardized personality inventory into our instructional system in the COURSEWRITER language, we not only attain automatic test administration and scoring through the use of counters, but data collection on reaction times as well. While only 25 students have taken the test to date, some anecdotal observations seem to suggest that the latency measures are more sagacious than the overt scoring procedure. Eventually, the personality variables might be used in individual sequencing of course presentation through the analytic power of the computer.

The many uses of CAI for research and development can only be suggested from our work and its interpretation. It will be for further studies and discussion to suggest more imaginative uses for available technology in order to meet our educational goals.

References

1. Grubb, R. E. and Selfridge, Lenore. "The Computer Tutoring of Statistics," *Computers and Automation,* March 1964, pp. 20-26.

2. Grubb, R. E. "The Effects of Paired Student Interaction in the Computer Tutoring of Statistics," paper read at national convention of the National Society for Programmed Instruction, Philadelphia, May 1965.

3. IBM Systems Reference Library Manual, "Computer Assisted Instruction—IBM 1401, 1440 or 1460 Operating System," Form C24-3253-1.

4. Schurdak, John. "An Approach to the Use of Computers in the Instructional Process and an Evaluation," IBM Research Center Report, RC-1432.

5. Uttal, W. R., Charap, M., and Maher, A. "The Computer Tutoring of Stenotype: a preliminary report," IBM Research Center Report, RC-724.

Part VI

Summary and Perspective

In order to provide a framework for considering and relating the papers in this Proceedings, Stolurow suggests a general strategy for educational technology based on feedback to the innovator so that changed instructional processes can be objectively evaluated—rather than accepted or discarded on subjective grounds.

Following the presentation of general strategy, there is a point-by-point consideration of many fine points of programming technique, research, and utilization in which the author goes to the papers presented at the Conference for examples and suggestions.

Summary and Perspective

LAWRENCE M. STOLUROW, Ph.D.*

The ferment in medical education revealed by the papers and discussions of the last two and one-half days is most encouraging to me both as a psychologist with a professional commitment to the study of learning and as a private citizen who is a consumer of medical services. Like all fermentation, however, it can result in either a delicious brew or a sour, unpotable liquid. The problem is to keep the conditions favorable to the production of the brew, and, if possible, to catalyze its activity.

Before focusing on the fine grain of the ferment as revealed here, let me make some points about the general strategy of educational technology which seem relevant. Later, I shall want to say a few things about the future.

General Strategy

Both Deterline and Mager, for example, have referred to the need to provide feedback to the program developer. In the early stages of innovation, this feedback to the innovator is a critical problem. He needs diagnostically useful feedback, however. While more innovations are *ineffective* than the reverse, it is generally true that there is *some* merit in many innovations. The problem, therefore, lies in finding those aspects which are effective, so they can be separated out from the counterbalancing ineffective factors with

*Professor of Psychology and Educational Psychology, University of Illinois, Champaign, Illinois.

which they are combined. Tests given at the end of a program which simply provide a global evaluation, or an over-all appraisal, rather than a detailed analysis of the effects produced by both the new and the old methods, are insufficient and wasteful. The student performance in which we are interested is both compound and complex, and an over-all evaluation simply tells us about the total score. It does not relate specific parts of the student's performance to the behavioral objectives of the program. We need to know—for each objective—whether the program was a failure or success. My *first* point about strategy is that any test used to assess the effects of a program needs to be developed as carefully as the program itself. My *second* point is that the post-test needs to measure, at a minimum, the objectives of the program as they were identified in the task analysis. My third point is that the test should also measure more particularly the transfer of training.

One reason that Mager's "learner-controlled" procedure is so useful is that it provides the program developer with a fine grain view of the learning process he is producing with his materials. It makes things visible to the programmer that otherwise might not come to light. In particular, one gets a view of the logic of instructional sequences which different learners seem to require.

While Lloyd's use of the structured interview provides informational feedback to the programmer, the information comes retrospectively. Therefore, it is not as useful for data about the sequence of frames as Mager's learner-controlled procedure. Its value should not, however, be overlooked in a complete developmental effort.

FINE GRAIN

In considering some of the fine grain of the ferment dealt with in these papers, my remarks will range over several topics. The first is sequence and ability.

Sequence and Ability

It is important for us, as programmers of educational materials, to learn more about sequential requirements of learners. This is one of the most neglected but interesting pedagogical questions confronting us.

Learning theory is silent on this problem, for it has focused upon the identification of two necessary and sufficient conditions: *contiguity* and *reinforcement*. Stimuli sequence, while obviously critical to the efficient learning and retention of knowledge and skills, is neither extensively studied nor well understood.

A content expert, on the other hand, often would lead you to believe that there is only *one* logical development to his subject matter. Furthermore, the organization he will suggest will be that of the sophisticated and knowledgeable expert. Actually, what the expert is describing is a *terminal,* not a beginning organization. Examination of texts reveals that experts often differ in their organization of topics, and task analyses of terminal performance will quickly reveal that few subject matter areas have necessary priorities built into them, that there are many different ways in which topics and frame sequences within these can be organized.

My point here is that there is not *just one* logical organization to a subject matter; there are many logical arrangements. What we need to find is *not the logical sequence,* but rather *the psychological sequence.* Furthermore, it is not one sequence for all learners, it is a set of sequences each of which is [may be] most efficient for a particular learner [group of learners].

The search for the principles that provide guidance for the psychological sequence to use for a learner is not without its hazards, however. A common practice in program development is to look for *the* sequence by determining the errors made by all students with whom the program is used. Typically this is done with a very small number of students. This use of a small number of uncharacterized learners is an inefficient and dangerous procedure.

It is *inefficient* as a basis for generalization to all students in that it is most likely to lead you to revise frames that don't really need to be revised for the group at large. In other words, if you see a 5 percent error rate as your minimum level, and use just 5 students, then every frame missed by one student gets revised. Particularly, if no record is kept of the type of student used, then it may be assumed that they are all alike. We have found that if you use such a small sample to represent all students and check the decision you make against a larger, more representative set such as 100 students, then very few of the frames that were judged to be bad when only 5 students were used, actually exceeded the 5 percent level when 100 students were used (see Frinke and Stolurow, 1965). If a program is being prepared for general use, then you should use a sample of such size [sample of sufficient size should be used such] that at least *two* students have to make an error on one frame in order for it to exceed your minimum error rate. If, for example, you use as a minimum a 10 percent level, then you should use at least 20 students. Preferably, however, the number should be even greater than a multiple of two if you believe in individual differences. I hope you will believe that there are real individual differences after hearing some of my later remarks.

The procedure of using a small number of students also is *dangerous* because in revising frames based upon error rate, it is more likely that the revised program will have more steps than are needed by all students, or even by the majority of students. Therefore, it is more likely to be boring to a large number, or at least more time-consuming than is necessary or desirable. Consequently, the best students are apt to dislike it. This procedure is likely to bias the development programs of program favoring the poorer student.

This brings us to the next point, which is that more than one set of materials and sequences seems to be required to optimize the learning of large groups of students. One way in which this argument for selective sampling and branching is revealed is through the relationships between particular learner characteristics such as mathematical ability, verbal ability, memory or reasoning, and the achievement test scores obtained after students have worked with different sequences of the same frames. These correlations reveal that the rank order of the students on the achievement test can change as a result of being exposed to different sequences of the *same* set of frames (Smith, 1962; Cartwright, 1962). This strongly suggests that the particular sequences one uses will determine the aptitudes and skills that an individual must use to master the subject matter.

There is a fitting analogy in the relation between the objective of a program and the objective of a trip. In both the program and the trip some means is required to get to a distant point. If in taking a trip, the members of a group are asked to *run* to a distant point (the objective), then the fastest runners will get there first. If, however, the same group is required to reach the same distant point by *swimming,* then the fastest swimmers will get there first. Similarly, if the instructional program is so organized that one merely has to *remember* previously presented material in order to understand a point being made by a frame, then the students with the best memories will get the point. However, if the instructional program requires *reasoning* in the form of relating two or more things not explicitly connected for them, then those with the highest reasoning aptitude will make the best scores.

This point can be related to the Wilds and Zachert paper, for example. They report in their interesting study that "The results for the academic year 1964-65 indicate that when conventional multiple-choice testing is used, there is little difference in the performance of control and experimental groups . . . " They conclude from this that ". . . the applications text did not significantly alter the student's learning of 'content'." From my point of view, it is quite possible that the use of the applications text resulted in a different rank order of students without changing the average performance of the group. In other words, it is possible that the use of the applications text affected the performance of students who were high in aptitude X and resulted in their achieving top scores while *not* changing the group mean, because those low in X earned low scores.

Anderson, Owen, and Hall (1965) also report data on the relationship between student characteristics and the effectiveness of different teaching methods. They report that "Women appeared to learn better from the lectures, men from the program, and those students whose native language was other than English benefited more from programmed instruction than from the lectures. Finally . . . teaching programme was also more effective than even the very carefully prepared lectures for the academically weak student." It is not necessary to assume that the match between these student characteristics and either the programs or the lectures would always be as described here. Rather, given two or more methods of teaching the same objectives, those methods will differ in their effectiveness with students who have different characteristics.

If this hypothesis is useful, then it has methodological implications for studies using different instructional methods or programs in medical schools. To test the hypothesis, the research design should include, as a pretest, a battery of ability tests, so that each of them can be correlated with the student's achievement and attitude scores after each method of instruction. By implication, different ones of these tests will correlate significantly with the achievement test scores under the different methods.

Confirmation of this ability-method hypothesis would mean that the way to *increase* the group's average post-test score would be to use each method in such a way as to achieve a match between the aptitude of an individual learner and the aptitude requirements of the method. Having done this it should be possible to raise the group average, since every student would be taught by that method which maximized his performance.

MULTIPLE CRITERIA

A related point concerns the use of multiple criteria in the evaluation of alternative programs. In the literature, it has been reported that prompting, for example, has led to more rapid learning than confirmation, but that confirmation led to better retention (Stolurow and Lippert, 1965). This finding raises a question about the priority to be given to various criteria. Obviously, when different methods produce different effects, one method might be used if an effect such as rapid learning is wanted, whereas a different method should be used if another effect, for example retention, is more important. Fortunately, in another study, it was found that by using prompting *first,* at a *lower* criterion level of performance, and then using confirmation, it was possible to get both rapid learning and better retention. This possibility of developing a *hybrid* method that optimizes a set of criteria may not always exist. If it does not, a decision will have to be made among the objectives and the desired effects.

Dr. Manning's paper touched on this point when he reported that his programmed lecture took longer to cover a given amount of material than did a regular lecture. He indicated that the programmed lecture resulted in student achievement at a higher level of problem-solving than had been achieved by conventional lectures. In other words, to get the problem-solving behavior it was necessary to use a method that required slower learning. It seems that we may have to decide which criterion we want. This same decision may be necessary in choosing between learning outcomes and attitude. Hopefully, decisions of this type will be optimized when we have greater knowledge of the variables involved.

ATTITUDE TOWARD INSTRUCTION

Several studies sought measures of student attitude toward programming (e.g., Lloyd, Anderson, Owen, and Hall). In general, the students seem to like the programmed learning experience. While this result is gratifying, it could provide more useful data had a standardized attitude instrument been developed. Then that same instrument could be used to obtain data from many different schools and courses and the results could be compared. A related point is that it might have been helpful to obtain both pre- and post-test attitude scores in order to determine what changes took place.

MEASUREMENT OF GAIN

Mager and Richardson concerned themselves with the evaluation problem. Change in student behavior is acknowledged as a desirable measure of learning, but change is not nearly so easy to determine in interpretable form as we would like. If all students started out at the same level, then a simple difference score would be meaningful. However, if they do not, as is frequently the case, then problems arise. Mager suggested using an index of the percentage gained by the student in relation to the maximum gain he could have secured (modified gain index). Another measure is one that is called a *regression score*. It is obtained by correlating the pretest with the post-test scores and then obtaining for each student the difference between his predicted post-test score and his actual post-test score. With this score, discrepancies from the expected score become the index of the effectiveness of the program.

NATURE OF CRITERION AND OBJECTIVES

Richardson's argument for the use of what the physician actually does in the care of patients as a learning criterion is very much to the point. However, the "specialist criterion performance" as I understand it, is not merely a behavioral standard for testing, it also constitutes a task analysis and provides an operational specification for the obectives of the program. I'm sorry, but I was not able to identify the error in the flow chart; but in spite of the error, the fact that the chart was done is most commendable. This analysis of the final performance is very important and useful.

REINFORCEMENT—delayed vs. immediate

One of the more interesting findings was in the paper by Lloyd, in which he reported that "Nine out of ten students chose the method using *delayed* feedback as being both more effective and preferred." It would be most interesting to know if this result would hold up under replication. It cannot be accepted with confidence, however, until data are secured on more students and the delayed and immediate feedback are used on different halves of the same subject matter. Unfortunately, content and procedure were confounded in this particular design to such an extent that we must look to further experimentation for definitive answers.

WASHBACK PROCEDURE

Lang, Paulson and Scott reported that they used a washback procedure in their dental anatomy program. One of the questions raised in a recent study by Merrill (1963) concerns the desirability of using washback on correction procedure. Merrill found that when he employed it, the students learned no more than when he did not use it. However, he did find that with the washback procedure the students took more time per frame and per test item. It seemed to make them more cautious without teaching them more.

VARIABLE FRAME SIZE

Garrett has raised a question about size of step or the size of the student's "operant span." This problem has reappeared over the years and is in need of solution. While we cannot solve it here, it is obvious to all of us that students can and do learn now, reading frames that are as long as a book. Seldom do we read a book "in one bite." With a book, the student determines his own size of bite, however, and this tends to increase as he becomes a better reader.

It is possible that instructions could be given to the reader in the margin of a book after each paragraph, so that no matter where he stops, he could test himself. We now have texts that provide questions after each chapter and some that also provide the answers. However, the author has made the frame a chapter long and uniform for all learners. It might be far better to allow for a wide variety of stopping points with continuing opportunity for feedback and confirmation.

PERSPECTIVE

Some points that might contribute to the focus of interest and activity in the future seem indicated, particularly in view of questions raised by these several papers.

MACHINE PRESENTATION VS. PROGRAM ALONE

People frequently behave as if "hardware" produced some unique effect. Studies comparing the effectiveness of linear programs presented by a machine, with their effectiveness when presented without one, have not shown an advantage for the machine mode. This result seems predictable when we consider the comparison in terms of the *functions* generally performed by these machines. A functional analysis, as performed in a systems approach to instruction, seems to be a useful way of looking at this pedagogical problem. From this point of view, the group which worked without the machine performed functions for themselves that the machine performed for the others. Essentially, the machine turned pages for the student.

In general terms, functional analysis suggests that machines can only be expected to contribute to the student's achievement when they perform a unique function, or perform a common function significantly more efficiently than it can be performed by students engaged in learning.

COMPUTER-ASSISTED INSTRUCTION

This leads to the question of CAI, about which Geis and Grubb have reported. The early uses of computers as central processing units for a teaching machine did not add new functions to those performed by simpler equipment. As a result, the findings clearly indicated that one could use a computer to teach, but little was added to our knowledge about the technology of instruction. Following these early efforts, there have been some major steps forward. In fact, it is now possible to do with computers things we cannot do by other means.

SOCRATES—an acronym for System for Organized Content to Review and Teach Educational Subjects—is a CAI facility in our laboratory that is now almost two years old. It has been used for over 1500 student hours.

Basically, this system performs three *sets* of functions: (1) Pre-tutorial functions; (2) tutorial functions; and (3) teacher-substitution functions. All these functions are carried out for each student, under student-paced conditions. Each student's record, in terms of aptitude, personality, and beginning information, is read into the system and used in making decisions about the teaching strategy to be used and the implementation of strategy when it is in use. In other words, SOCRATES uses a set of rules for making decisions specifically related to each individual student, depending upon that student's characteristics in relation to given teaching objectives. In addition, the strategy or set of rules is changed in the process of teaching the student if his responses reveal that he is not performing up to expectation on the protocol.

Let me make these processes more explicit: The information

which the pretest battery reveals about a particular student is stored and is used in making decisions about the learning mode. His aptitude scores determine the sequence, and his personality scores determine the nature of the evaluative feedback he sees after making each response. An aggressive student, for example, may see only negative statements when he makes wrong responses. For example, "That is a terrible response, you can do better than that." The decision to use this teaching rule to provide a program that "fights back" would be in conformity with findings obtained by Frase (1963). In a way, they represent the type of thing Howard was referring to in his paper—namely, introducing some of the teacher's personality into the instructional material. The CAI system, however, can introduce several different teacher personalities, depending upon the student's personality characteristics. Furthermore, the student can indicate whether he wants to change the teacher or not. He can be evaluated for correct and incorrect responses or neither whenever he chooses.

In addition, instructional rules can be changed by the system itself while the student is being taught. If a student's latency is too long, he may be given frames at a simpler level. If he responds correctly to a set of frames, he may be shipped to a new concept.

In addition, the computer is used to author programs. Given sentence forms, word-lists and rules, it can write a linear program. It can generate problems like syllogisms which the student uses in learning to apply the rules of validity. These routines permit the use of the system in an ever-adaptive fashion, since the number of problems can be adjusted to each student's needs as determined by his proficiency level.

SUMMARY

The conference papers are an impressive demonstration of sincerity and concern for the improvement of medical education. They suggest a vigorous and rapidly approaching maturity. While the research efforts have not all been equally successful, they have been encouraging. They may have taught the programmers more than the students, but this is not to be discounted in its general effect. The efforts should be looked at in terms of the realtime line—for skill in implementing a new technology develops slowly. A further complication stems from the fact that the technology itself is maturing, so that the mastery of linear programming skills leads naturally to the development of skills in writing branching programs, and, finally, to the preparation of CAI materials. This is a transition, not a liquidation process. Branching and linear programs can be used in a CAI system, and the decision functions which the computer can contribute can be added once the prime educational program is available.

It would be desirable now to use the medical aptitude scores of students in correlation studies of achievement under different instructional conditions. In this way, it will be possible to realize more fully the potential of self-instruction as a truly individualized educational approach. The conference papers indicate that there is a substantial development leading in this direction in medical education. I hope it continues to full fruition.

References

1. Cartwright, G. P. "Two-Types of Programmed Instruction for Mentally Retarded Adolescents" Unpublished Master's thesis, University of Illinois, 1962. (Abstracted in Schramm, W. *The Research on Programmed Instruction*. Washington, D. C.: Office of Education, OE 34034, No. 35. 1964).

2. Frase, L. T. "Experimental Analysis of Three Patterns of Presenting a Standard Logic Task." Urbana, Illinois: University of Illinois, Training Research Laboratory USOE Title VII. Project No. 2-20-003. Quarterly Report No. 6. 1963.

3. Stolurow, L. M., & Lippert, H., "Prompting, Confirmation, and Overlearning in the Automated Teaching of a Sight Vocabulary." In J. P. DeCecco (Ed.), *Educational Technology: Readings in Programmed Instruction*. New York: Holt, Rinehart and Winston, 1964.

4. Merrill, M. D. "Learning and Retention of a Model and a Preview in Teaching an Imaginary Science." Urbana Illinois: University of Illinois, Training Research Laboratory. Contract 2-20-003, November, 1963. Technical Report No. 3.

5. Smith, L. M. "Programmed Learning in Elementary School: An Experimental Study of Relationships Between Mental Abilities and Performance." Urbana, Illinois: University of Illinois, 1962, *mimeo.* (Abstracted in Schramm, W. *The Research on Programmed Instruction*. Washington, D. C.: Office of Education, OE 34034, No. 35. 1964).

6. Frinke, G. and Stolurow, L. M. "A Study of Sample Size in Making Decisions about Instructional Materials." *Educational and Psychological Measurement*. Vol. 26, No. 3 (Autumn) 1966.

Note: Within the context of the paper, Professor Stolurow refers to the following authors' articles found in this text:

a. Anderson, Owen, Hall and Smart, pp. 114-130
b. Deterline, pp. 33-39
c. Lloyd, pp 138-147
d. Mager, pp 40-53
e. Richardson, pp. 54-61
f. Wilds and Zachert, pp. 84-101

Bibliography

General References

Austwick, Kenneth (ed.): *Teaching Machines and Programming*. New York: Macmillan Co., 1964.
A symposium of papers relating the early research efforts of British workers in the field of programmed instruction.

Becker, James L.: *A Programmed Guide to Writing Auto-Instructional Programs*. Camden, N. J.: RCA Service Company, 1963.
An attempt to combine some instructions on constructing a program with a model self-instructional course.

Bloom, Benjamin S., *et al.: Taxonomy of Educational Objectives—The Classification of Educational Goals: Handbook I: The Cognitive Domain*. New York: Longmans, Green, 1956.
A very useful reference for the development of behavioral goals for instruction; the handbook provides many examples as well as a rationale.

Brethower, Dale M.: *Programmed Instruction: A Manual of Programming Techniques*. Chicago: Educational Methods, 1963.
A linear program designed to teach some fundamental aspects of program writing.

Brethower, Dale M., Markle, D. G., Rummler, G. A., Schrader, A. W., and Smith, D. E. P.: *Programmed Learning: A Practicum*. Ann Arbor, Mich.: Ann Arbor Publishers, 1965.
A programmed introduction to programming, including examples of good and poor frames, effective and ineffective sequences.

Coulson, John E. (ed.): *Programmed Learning and Computer-Based Instruction*. New York: John Wiley & Sons, 1962.
Proceedings of the conference on application of digital computers to automated instruction. This volume is the first effort to couple in systematic fashion the developments in learning methodology with computer technology.

De Cecco, John P. (ed.): *Educational Technology*. New York: Holt, Rinehart, and Winston, 1964.
A collection of papers and research reports on programmed instruction. Particularly useful are the grouped studies on such program variables as the stimulus, the response, and feedback.

Deterline, William A.: *An Introduction to Programmed Instruction*. Englewood Cliffs, N. J.: Prentice-Hall, 1962.
A brief orientation to the subject designed for the general reader.

Dolmatch, Theodore B., Marting, Elizabeth, and Finley, Robert E. (ed.): *Revolution in Training: Programmed Instruction in Industry*. New York: American Management Association, 1962.
While this volume deals primarily with industrial and business training, its implications for adult and paramedical education are evident. Contains many case histories of utilization.

Filep, Robert T. (ed.): *Prospectives in Programming*. New York: Macmillan Co., 1963.
A collection of papers that represent lectures presented at several summer institutes on programmed instruction under the auspices of the Center for Programmed Instruction.

Fine, Benjamin: *Teaching Machines*. New York: Sterling, 1962.
A popularized, non-technical introduction to self-instruction, with personalized reactions of the author to programs, devices, and the use of self-instruction.

Fry, Edward B.: *Teaching Machines and Programmed Instruction*. New York: McGraw-Hill, 1963.
An introduction to the theory of, and research on, programmed instruction. This volume is designed for the reader who wants detailed orientation to the subject.

Galanter, Eugene (ed.): *Automatic Teaching: The State of the Art*. New York: John Wiley & Sons, 1959.
This volume ranks as one of the historic firsts in the field, and presents a series of early research and speculative papers.

Glaser, Robert (ed.): *Teaching Machines and Programmed Learning, II: Data and Directions*. Washington, D. C.: National Education Association, 1965.
A companion volume to Lumsdaine and Glaser cited below. A series of papers taking a detailed look at what has been accomplished in the five years following the appearance of the first source book on programmed instruction.

Green, Edward J.: *The Learning Process and Programmed Instruction*. New York: Holt, Rinehart, and Winston, 1962.
Primarily a treatment of the theoretical aspects of learning and the experimental basis for programmed instruction.

Hendershot, Carl H. (ed.): *Programmed Learning: A Bibliography of Programs and Presentation Devices*. (Offset) University Center, Michi-

gan: Delta College (Quarterly).
The most complete, and most frequently updated, bibliography of available programs and self-instructional devices.

Holtz, Herman R., and Alter, Paul A.: *A Short Course in Intrinsic Programming*. Silver Spring, Md.: U. S. Industries, 1965.
A short branching program designed to introduce the student to planning and constructing branching sequences.

Hughes, John L.: *Programmed Instruction for Schools and Industry*. Chicago: Science Research Associates, 1962.
An early effort to describe programming with some consideration to the construction of a programmed sequence.

Hughes, John L.: *Programmed Learning: A Critical Evaluation*. Chicago: Educational Methods, 1963.
Reports of program utilization with adult learners, followed by discussions of participating psychologists and educators.

Jacobs, Paul I., Maier, Milton H. and Stolurow, Lawrence M.: *A Guide to Evaluating Self-Instructional Programs*. New York: Holt, Rinehart, and Winston, 1966.
A brief and simply written discussion of points to be considered in selecting and evaluating learning programs.

Judge, Richard D., and Romano, Michael T.: *Health Science Television: A Review*. Ann Arbor, Michigan: University of Michigan Medical Center, 1965.
A selection of papers from the 7th Annual Meeting of The Council on Medical Television.

Keller, Fred S.: *Learning: Reinforcement Theory*. New York: Random House, 1954.
Perhaps the briefest, and most readable, exposition of the reinforcement theory of learning on which programming is based.

Krathwohl, David A., *et al.: Taxonomy of Educational Objectives— The Classification of Educational Goals: Handbook II: Affective Domain*. New York: David McKay, 1964.
A continuation of the development and exemplification of objective goals for instruction. See *Bloom* above.

Leedham, John and Unwin, Derek (eds): *Aspects of Educational Technology*. London: Methuen, 1967.
The Proceedings of the Programmed Learning Conference held at Loughborough in 1966. Contributed papers from research workers in England and other countries.

Lindvall, C. M. (ed.): *Defining Educational Objectives*. A report of the Regional Commission on Educational Coordination and the Learning Research and Development Center. Pittsburgh: University of Pittsburgh Press (Paperback), 1964.
A careful examination of the process of specifying educational goals, and its application to programmed instruction, the general learning process, and curriculum design.

Lumsdaine, Arthur A., and Glaser, Robert (eds.): *Teaching Machines and Programmed Learning*. Washington, D. C.: National Education Association, 1960.
A valuable source book that collects the significant papers on programmed instruction from 1926 to 1960.

Lysaught, Jerome P. (ed.): *Programmed Learning*. Ann Arbor, Mich.: Foundation for Research on Human Behavior, 1961.
An early collection of papers by Skinner, Lumsdaine, and others addressed to the implications of programming for adult education.

Lysaught, Jerome P. (ed.): *Programmed Instruction in Medical Education*. Rochester, N. Y.: The University of Rochester, 1965.
Proceedings of the First Rochester Conference on Programmed Instruction in Medical Education. An analytic treatment of self-instruction, with reports on initial research and application of programs to medical teaching.

Lysaught, Jerome P., and Williams, Clarence M.: *A Guide to Programmed Instruction*. New York: John Wiley, 1963.
A general text on the planning and construction of programmed sequences. A step-by-step process is developed and illustrated. A Yugoslavian edition is available. German, Spanish, and other editions are in press.

Mager, Robert F.: *Preparing Objectives for Programmed Instruction*. San Francisco: Fearon, 1961.
A brief, well-designed program on the construction and phrasing of behavioral goals for use in programmed learning.

Margulies, Stuart, and Eigen, Lewis D.: *Applied Programmed Instruction*. New York: John Wiley & Sons, 1962.
A collection of papers and research reports on applications of programmed learning to adult learning situations.

Markle, Susan M.: *Good Frames and Bad*. New York: John Wiley & Sons, 1964.
A useful programmed grammar of frame writing designed to aid the reader in writing items for various program models, and in editing items according to selected principles of programming.

Nunney, Derek N. (ed.): *New Approaches in Educational and Training Systems*. Detroit: Wayne State University, 1965. (Offset.)
A collection of papers relating to educational systems and self-instruction with emphasis on the adult learner.

Ofiesh, Gabriel D.: *Programmed Instruction: A Guide to Management*. New York: American Management Association, 1965.
A collection of reports and case studies on the applications of self-instruction to business and industry training situations. Includes one chapter on professional education with examples drawn from medicine.

Ofiesh, Gabriel D., and Meierhenry, Wesley C. (eds.): *Trends in Pro-*

grammed Instruction. Washington, D. C.: National Education Association, 1964.
The Proceedings of the first national convention of the National Society for Programmed Instruction.

Pierleoni, Robert G. (ed): *Perspectives in Programming.* Rochester, N. Y.: Genesee Valley Programming Society and The University of Rochester, 1967. Proceedings of a conference on programmed instruction in the sixties with a series of papers on the use of self-instruction in health education, particularly nursing instruction.

Pipe, Peter: *Practical Programming.* New York: Holt, Rinehart & Winston, 1965.
A very brief introduction to the construction and development of programmed learning sequences.

Plym, Alberta, and Aikawa, Jerry K.: *The Evaluation of Laboratory Data by Means of Quality Control.* Denver, Colo.: Central Laboratory, University of Colo. Medical Center, 1965.
A programmed Instruction Manual which won an award for instructional innovation in 1965.

Programmed Instruction and the Hospital. Chicago, Ill.: Hospital Research and Educational Trust, 1967.
Proceedings of an institute held jointly by the Trust and Teachers College, Columbia University exploring the applications and implications of programmed instruction for the continuing educational needs of hospitals and other health facilities.

Roucek, Joseph S. (ed.): *Programmed Teaching: A Symposium of Automation in Education.* New York: Philosophical Library, 1965.
A recent collection of papers related to the application of self-instruction to various subject-matter fields.

Russell, William O. and Kolvoord, Robert A. (eds): *Education for Tomorrow: Developments in Educational Technology.* Chicago, Ill.: American Society for Clinical Pathologists, 1966.
A collection of papers designed to explore the requirements of continuing education programs for the medical specialties, and to suggest steps to be taken for the improvement of individualized and self-instruction of physicians.

Schramm, Wilber (ed.): *The Research on Programmed Instruction.* Washington, D. C.: Office of Education, 1964 (OE-34034).
An annotated bibliography of research on programmed instruction reported between 1955 and 1962.

Smith, Wendell I., and Moore, James W. (eds.): *Programmed Learning.* New York: D. Van Nostrand Co., 1962.
A short collection of the early, significant papers in the field, coupled with a few selected research studies.

Stolurow, Lawrence M.: *Teaching by Machine.* Washington, D. C.: Office of Education, 1961 (OE-34010).
A distillation of early research studies and speculative papers.

Taber, Julian I., Glaser, Robert, and Shaefer, Halmuth H.: *Learning and Programmed Instruction*. Reading, Mass.: Addison-Wesley, 1965.
An introduction to the theory and principles of programmed instruction, with a discussion and examples of techniques for programming material.

Teal, Gilbert (ed.): *Programmed Instruction in Industry and Education*. Stamford, Conn.: Public Service Research, 1963.
Proceedings of the first institute devoted to the application of programmed instruction to adult learning.

Thomas, C. A., Davies, I. K., Openshaw, D., and Bird, J. B.: *Programmed Learning in Perspective*. Chicago: Educational Methods, 1964.
A guide to the development and construction of self-instructional programs using a matrix system developed in England.

Varty, Jonathan: *Collegiate Programmed Instruction*. (mimeo.). New York: Brooklyn College.
A regularly revised bibliography of available programs designed for college-level instruction. (Publication currently suspended.)

Walther, Richard E., and Crowder, Norman A.: *Techniques in Intrinsic Programming*. Silver Spring, Md.: U. S. Industries, Inc., 1965.
A guide to the writing of branching or intrinsic programs based primarily on the requirements of the Autotutor teaching device.

Journals

Audio-Visual Instruction. Washington, D. C.: Department of Audio-Visual Instruction, National Education Association.

Audio-Visual Communication Review. Washington, D. C.: Department of Audio-Visual Instruction, National Education Association.

Bulletin of the Clearinghouse on Self-Instructional Materials for Health Care Facilities. Rochester, N. Y.: Rochester Clearinghouse, The University of Rochester.

Contemporary Psychology. Washington, D. C.: American Psychological Association.

Journal of the National Society for Programmed Instruction. San Antonio, Texas: NSPI, Trinity University.

Journal of Programmed Instruction. New York: Institute of Educational Technology, Teachers College, Columbia University. (Publication suspended June 1966)

Programmed Instruction. (Bulletin) New York: Institute of Educational Technology, Teachers College, Columbia University. (Publication suspended June 1966)

Teaching Aids News. Saddle Brook, N. J.: Educational News Service. (Now published under the title: *Educational Technology*.)

Articles on Medical Programming

Allender, Jerome S.: The programming of instructional materials for medical education. *J. Med. Educ.* 39:346-354 (April) 1964.
A report of early programming activities in medicine and a discussion of the varied kinds of learning that might be affected by future programs.

Allender, Jerome S., Bernstein, Lionel M., and Miller, George E.: Differential achievement and differential cost in programmed instruction and conventional instruction in internal medicine. *J. Med. Educ.* 40: 825-831 (September) 1965.
Results and analysis of comparing standard texts, lectures, programmed texts, and teaching machines to teach renal function and renal failure at three medical schools.

Bridgman, Charles: A lecture response device: a preliminary report on a key aspect of a co-ordinated teaching program in anatomy. *J. Med. Educ.* 39:132-139 (February) 1964.
Report of a classroom communicator system adapted for use in teaching anatomy at The Univeristy of Kansas Medical Center. Employing stimulus, response, and feedback techniques, the system enhances the individual learning of the students while freeing the teacher from many manual classroom tasks.

Brown, Murray C.: Electronics and medical education. *J. Med. Educ.* 38:270-281 (April) 1963.
A discussion on the implications of computer technology for the future of medical education with emphasis on the probable changes in educational programs.

Can undergraduate or postgraduate medical education benefit from programmed instruction? Pfizer *Spectrum* 10:88-95 (Sept.-Oct.) 1962.
A brief introduction to the use of programs for medical education; the article includes a short sequence on EKG demonstrating how a program teaches.

Cheris, Barbara H.: On comparing programming and other teaching methods. *J. Med. Educ.* 39:304-310 (March) 1964.
A brief review of the literature and a discussion of certain research studies in programmed instruction covering the period 1958-1963.

Cheris, Barbara H., and Cheris, David N.: Programmed instruction versus a textual presentation of radiology. *J. Med. Educ.* 39:311-318 (March) 1964.
Report of a controlled study of 46 medical students, one half of whom used a programmed text in radiology. Significant differences were recorded on post-tests and retention tests, with the program students demonstrating greater achievement.

Demone, Harold W., and Spiegel, Allen D.: *Evaluation of an automated teaching machine program for continuing education of physicians.* Boston: Medical Foundation, 1963.

Use of a program and teaching machine for practitioners; learning was achieved, but difficulties in time and motivation were observed in a limited study situation.

Dryer, Bernard V.: Thinking men and thinking machines in medicine. *J. Med. Educ.* 38:82-89 (February) 1963.

A discussion of aspects of computer technology for medical education, with particular emphasis on learning and thinking. A reflection of possible promises and problems to come with increased machine efficiency.

Eaton, M. T., Strough, L. C., and Muffly, R. B.: Programmed instruction in basic psychopathology. *J. Med. Educ.* 39:86-89 (January) 1964.

Report of a pilot study using 20 students. Results in terms of achievement and efficiency were encouraging to further exploration of programming in medical education.

Elder, S. T., Meckstroth, G. R., Nice, C. M., Jr., and Meyers, P. H.: A comparison of a linear program in radiation with traditional lecture presentation of the same material. *J. Med. Educ.* 39:1078-1082 (December) 1964.

A brief report on two experiments using a program with 36 medical students and 16 technicians. The program performed as well as the conventional lecture for the medical students, its intended population. Results indicated modifications would be required for the technicians.

Entwisle, George, and Entwisle, D. R.: The use of a digital computer as a teaching machine. *J. Med. Educ.* 39:802-812 (October) 1963.

A brief report on the use of a program combined with a computer to teach diagnosis. Possibilities are indicated for a high degree of individual adaptation coupled with an effective simulator by the storage facilities afforded by the computer.

Felson, B., Spitz, H. B., and Weinstein, A.: Programmed learning in radiology; a preliminary evaluation (abstract). *J. Med. Educ.* 38:786 (September) 1963.

Report of a limited study on matched halves of a junior class in radiology; learning was achieved, but retention of the program was not as great as that of a lecture. Questions for further research are raised.

Feurzeig, W., Munter, P., and Swets, J.: Computer-aided teaching in medical diagnosis. *J. Med. Educ.* 39:746-754 (August) 1964.

A description of a computer teaching program designed to assist in the instruction of medical diagnosis. A sample computer run is included as one illustration of the system.

Gildenberg, Robert F.: Student Retention of a Programmed Instruction Course in Immunohematology. *J. Med. Educ.* 42:62-68 (January) 1967.

Presentation of data collected while testing a program instruction course. Also, included are comments made by the students and recommendations for more effective administration of programs.

Graves, G. O. and Ingersol, R. W.: Comparison of learning attitudes. *J. Med. Educ.* 39:100-111 (February) 1964.

Report of a study of two groups of medical students taught anatomy by traditional methods and by experimental approaches emphasizing self-learning and self-direction. On traditional examinations, there was no significant difference in achievement. On examinations to test critical thinking, however, the experimental group was significantly superior.

Green, Edward J., and Weiss, Robert J.: Programmed instruction: for what, for whom, and how? *J. Med. Educ.* 38:264-269 (April) 1963.
An early discussion of the problems, promises, and inherent possibilities of programmed instruction in connection with medical education.

Green, E. J., Weiss, R. J., and Nice, P. O.: Experimental use of a programmed text in a medical school course. *J. Med. Educ.* 37:767-775 (August) 1962.
Report of a controlled study using a programmed text in parasitology. Both achievement and efficiency were demonstrably higher among students using the program.

Greenhill, Leslie P.: Communication research and the teaching-learning process. *J. Med. Educ.* 38:495-502 (June) 1963.
A review of research over a fifteen year period. Of particular interest is the discussion on the increased emphasis of developments related to self-instruction and individualized learning. Applications of the research to medical education are suggested.

Ham, T. Hale: The training of the physician: research in the teaching-learning process—Two Experimental Modules. *New Engl. J. Med.* 271:1042-1046 (November) 1964.
Two experimental programs are discussed, both designed to increase the self-instructional aspects of medical education. Emphasizes the increasingly important role of individual learning in medicine.

Hall, V. E.: Systematic use of immediate feedback in teaching physiology to medical students. *J. Med. Educ.* 39:1101-1106 (December) 1964.
A discussion of the importance and utility of rapid feedback in learning situations. A comparison of programmed instruction with conventional teaching in body fluid metabolism with improved results for the feedback (experimental) group.

Harless, William G. Development of a computer-assisted instruction program in a medical center environment. *J. Med. Educ.* 42:139-145 (February) 1967.
A discussion of "vocal programming" as a means to simplify and extend the use of computer-assisted programmed instruction in the university of Oklahoma Medical Center. A sample computer teaching sequence is included in the article.

Harris, J. W., Horrigan, D. L., Ginther, J. R., and Ham, T. H.: Pilot study in teaching hematology with emphasis on self-education by the students, *J. Med. Educ.* 37:719-736 (August) 1962.
Report of early trials of self-instructional materials in hematology. While not a program *per se,* the teaching materials were developed through a process similar to that employed in programming.

Hawkridge, David G., and Mitchell, David S.: Use of a programmed text during a course in genetics for medical students. *J. Med. Educ.* 42: 163-169 (February) 1967.
Discussion and results of the use of a programmed text on genetics with medical students at The University of Rhodesia. Achievement scores were at an acceptable level, and scores were more homogeneous at the end of instruction than at the beginning. Student reactions were favorable.

Huber, John Franklin: Programmed large group presentations. (abstract.) *J. Med. Educ.* 38:791 (September) 1963.
Report on an experimental approach using the concepts of programmed learning in television and film presentation.

Jason, Hilliard: Programmed instruction: new bottle of rediscovered wine. *Can. Med. Assn. Jour.* 92:711-716 (April 3) 1965.
An introductory paper on programmed instruction which seeks to relate its processes and potential to the larger field of teaching and learning.

Kirsch, A. D.: A medical training game using a computer as a teaching aid. *Meth. Inform. Med.* 2:138-143 (October) 1963.
A discussion of the development of a computer-assisted instructional program on diagnosis that would permit up to ten medical students to work simultaneously, but individually, through a presenting problem. There is hope that the system will have research possibilities in learning as well as instructional capability.

Lindberg, D. A.: A computer in medicine. *Missouri Med.* 61:282-284 (April) 1964.
Announcement of an acquisition of a computer for the Univeristy of Missouri Medical Center designed for aiding both the practice and teaching of medicine. There is a brief discussion of computers and medical education generally.

Lysaught, Jerome P.: Programmed instruction: a new departure in medical education. *New Phys.* 13:101-107 (April) 1964.
An orientation to programming in medical education, with a review of early research studies from 1962 to 1964.

Lysaught, Jerome P.: Programmed instruction for medical education: learner reactions to large-scale use. *New Phys.* 14:156-160 (June) 1965.
A presentation and analysis of reactions of more than 5,500 physicians and medical students to a programmed review of *Allergy and Hypersensitivity.*

Lysaught, Jerome P.: Self-instructional medical programs; a survey. *New Phys.* 13:52-55 (May) 1964.
A bibliographical listing of available and experimental programs in medical and paramedical fields.

Lysaught, Jerome P.: Self-instructional programs for continuing education. *Med. Times.* 93:978-989 (September) 1965.

A consideration of the implications of programmed learning for continuation education, with a number of examples of self-instructional sequences designed for various learning outcomes.

Lysaught, Jerome P.: The question: how to keep up? Partial answer: self-administered programmed instruction. *Resident Phys.* 12:135-160 (May) 1966.
A general article on the implications of programmed instruction for continuing education. Several sample programming sequences are shown to illustrate the varied capabilities of this self-instructional system.

Lysaught, Jerome P., and Jason, Hilliard: Programmed instruction in medical education: report of the Rochester conference: *J. Med. Educ.* 40:474-481 (May) 1965.
A brief summary of the papers and topics dealt with in the First Rochester Conference in Programmed Instruction in Medical Education.

Lysaught, Jerome P., Sherman, Charles D., Jr., and Williams, Clarence M.: Programmed learning: potential values for medical instruction. *JAMA* 189:803-807 (September 14) 1964.
A review of research together with a discussion of implications of programming for future medical education.

Martin, Donald S.: Teaching materials: CDC resources. *J. Med. Educ.* 39:32-38 (September) 1964.
Presentation on the kinds of teaching materials and aids that have been developed at the Communicable Disease Center with a plea for cooperative approaches in the future that would up-grade instruction on infectious diseases in the medical schools.

Meckstroth, G. R., Elder, S. T., Meyers, P. H., and Nice, C. M., Jr.: Programmed instruction in radiology at Tulane University School of Medicine. (offset, prepublication.) Available from authors.
A report of programming activities at Tulane with sample items from programs used to illustrate points in development.

Miller, G. E., Allender, J. S., and Wolf, A. V.: Differential achievement with programmed text, teaching machine, and conventional instruction in physiology. *J. Med. Educ.* 40:817-824 (September) 1965.
A discussion of branching programs for medical education, followed by the presentation and analysis of results using a program in body fluid metabolism at three medical schools. Self-instructional materials proved themselves to be both effective and efficient in terms of student learning.

Netsky, M. G., Banghart, F. W., and Hain, J. D.: Seminar versus lecture, and prediction of performance by medical students. *J. Med. Educ.* 39:112-119 (February) 1964.
Report of a controlled experiment comparing teacher-controlled and student-controlled learning modalities for medical students. While the

results are not definitive, they indicate promising possibilities for further research.

Owen, S. G.: A comparison of programmed instruction with conventional lectures in the teaching of final-year medical students. *J. Med. Educ.* 40:1058-1062 (November) 1965.
A series of tabular comparisons are presented on the teaching of electrocardiography to British medical students by means of a teaching machine program and a special lecture series.

Owen, S. G., Hall, R., Anderson, J., and Smart, G. A.: An experimental comparison of programmed instruction by teaching machine with conventional lecturing in the teaching of electrocardiography to final year medical students. London: *Postgrad. Med. J.* 41:201-206 (April) 1965.
An initial report and discussion on the research reported on this Second Rochester Conference.

Owen, S. G., Hall, R., and Waller, I. B.: Use of a teaching machine in medical education; preliminary experience with a programme in electrocardiography. London: *Postgrad. Med. J.* 59-65 (February) 1964.
Report on early field test experience with a branching program of 604 frames designed to teach ECG interpretation.

Peterson, Osler L.: Teaching diagnostic skills. *New Engl. J. Med.* 271:1046-1047 (November) 1964.
A discussion of the cooperative program in teaching hematology that places emphasis on the individualized, self-learning of the medical student.

Programmed learning in medical education. *Post-grad. Med. J.* 40:447 (August) 1964.
A short discussion of the applications of programmed instruction to medical education, including a consideration of the varieties of programming modalities and their probable effectiveness with medical learners.

Reynolds, Robert L.: A teaching tool for the health professions. *NSPI JOURNAL* 2:7-10 (December) 1963.
Some general observations on programming in medicine, followed by a description of the project at the Communicable Disease Center.

Ross, S. E.: Programmed instruction and medical education. *JAMA*. 182:938-39 (December) 1962.
An early discussion of the essential principles of programmed instruction, and the possible utility of the approach to medical instruction.

Spiegel, Allen D.: Evaluation of an automated teaching machine program for continuing education of physicians. *Mass. Gen. Pract. News* 13:12-14 (March) 1964.
A report of the reactions of 78 physicians who participated in a teaching machine course in the review of diabetes.

Terry, L. L.: The crisis in health communications. *Hospitals.* 38:49-51 (June) 1964.

Suggestion for greater use of skilled educational "middlemen" to work with technology, information theory, and other advances in the handling of the tremendous advances in knowledge coming out of research.

Warner, Homer R.: Medical diagnosis using a digital computer. *JAMA*. 181:293-322 (July) 1961.
Proceedings of the 3rd IBM Medical Symposium, includes a short discussion on the use of a computer to teach the diagnosis of congenital heart disease.

Weinshelbaum, A.: The use of a small, desk top analogue computer in nuclear medicine education. *J. Nucl. Med.* 5:58-68 (January) 1964.
Report of the use of small computer to instruct learners on hypothetical problems involving radioactive decay. Designed to teach concepts as well as specific problem-solving techniques.

Weiss, Robert J., and Green, E. J.: The applicability of programmed instruction in a medical school curriculum. *J. Med. Educ.* 37:760-766 (August) 1962.
A discussion of the possibilities for programmed instruction in medical education, and a brief description of the Dartmouth project intended to test those possibilities.

Programmed Units in Medicine

Ackerman, J. H., and Gilbert, T. F.: *Routine Epidemiological Investigation of Food-Borne Disease.* Atlanta, Georgia: USPHS Communicable Disease Center, 1963. Linear, mathetics program.

Allergy and Hypersensitivity, Third Edition, Revised. Developed jointly by Pfizer *Spectrum* and Basic Systems, Inc., New York: Chas. Pfizer & Co., Inc., 1966. Linear program. A Spanish edition has been prepared for Pfizer Spain by Dr. Luis Daufi.

Bernstein, L. M., Allender, J. S., Elstein, A. S., and Epstein, R. B.: *Renal Function and Renal Failure: A Programmed Text.* Baltimore: Williams & Wilkins, 1965. Branching program.

Campbell, Colin: *Anemias in Pregnancy.* (Field test edition.) Ann Arbor, Mich.: The University of Michigan Medical Center, 1965. Offset. Linear program.

Carnell, P. H., and Reusch, R. N.: *Molecular Equilibrium.* Philadelphia: W. B. Saunders Company, 1963. Linear program.

Carnell, P. H., and Reusch, R. N.: *Thermochemistry and Kinetics.* Philadelphia: W. B. Saunders Company, 1965. Linear program.

Cheris, David N., and Cheris, Barbara H.: *Basic Physics and Principles of Diagnostic Radiology.* Chicago: Year Book Medical Publishers, 1964. Linear program.

Christensen, Halvor N.: *Body Fluids and the Acid Base Balance.* Philadelphia: W. B. Saunders Company, 1964. Linear program.

Christensen, Halvor N., and Palmer, Graham A.: *Enzyme Kinetics.* Philadelphia: W. B. Saunders Co., 1966. Linear program for students.

Christensen, Halvor N.: *pH and Dissociation.* Philadelphia: W. B. Saunders Company, 1963. Linear program.

Cohen, J., Johnson, P., and Stolurow, L. M.: *Anatomy of the Trigeminal Nerve.* Urbana, Ill.: University of Illinois, 1965. Linear program. (Field test edition, offset.)

Coleman, R. D.: *Oral Anatomy in Local Anesthesia.* Department of Health, Education and Welfare (in press).

Current Concepts of Thyroid Disease. Developed jointly by Pfizer *Spectrum* and Basic Systems, Inc., New York: Chas. Pfizer & Co., Inc., 1965. Linear program.

Electrocardiography: The Arrythmias. Developed jointly by Warner-Chilcott Laboratories and Basic Systems, Inc., New York: Warner-Chilcott Laboratories, 1964. Linear program.

Endocrinology: Diagnosis and Treatment of Gynaecological Diseases. Developed jointly by The Crookes Laboratories Limited and Cambridge Consultants (Training) Limited. Basingstoke, Hampshire: The Crookes Laboratories Limited, 1965. Linear program in five booklets.

Felson, B., Weinstein, A., and Spitz, H.: *Principles of Chest Roentgenology.* Philadelphia: W. B. Saunders Company, 1965. Linear program.

Foy, J. M.: *The Mechanism of Urine Formation, Second Edition.* Bradford, England: The Bradford Institute of Technology, 1965. Branching program. (Field test edition, offset.)

Howard, John W.: *Using the Health Sciences Library: Part 1, The Card Catalog.* Morgantown, West Va.: Medical Center Library, The University of West Virginia, 1964. Branching program.

Immunohematology: Principles and Practice. Developed by Basic Systems, Inc. for Ortho Pharmaceutical Corp. New York: Ortho Pharmaceutical Corp., 1965. Linear program.

Ingram, I. M., and Mowbray, R. M.: *A Teaching Method and Refresher Course in the Affective Disorders.* London: Geigy Pharmaceuticals, Ltd., 1964. Linear program.

Kahn, Julius B.: *Autonomic Pharmacology: The Muscarinics and Adrenergics.* London, England: W. B. Saunders Ltd., 1966. Linear program for medical students.

Kessler, Edward, Cassamo, Leonard P., and Azneer, J. Leonard: *Diabetic Acidosis.* Los Angeles: Edlen Research, 1965. Linear program designed for use with self-instructional films.

Meckstroth, G. R., Elder, S. T., Nice, C. M., Jr., and Meyers, P. H.: *A Programmed Introduction to Radiation Protection.* New Orleans: Tulane University School of Medicine, 1964. Linear program.

Methods of Conception Control. Developed by Basic Systems, Inc. for Ortho Pharmaceutical Corp. New York: Ortho Pharmaceutical Corp., 1965. Linear program.

Meyers, Philip H., Roy, Manuel, Jr., and Nice, Charles M., Jr.: *Differential Diagnosis of Cardiovascular Disease by X-Ray*. New York, N.Y.: Harper & Row, 1966.

Nice, Charles M.: *Cardiovascular Roentgenology: A Validated Program*. New York, N.Y.: Harper & Row, 1967.

Nice, Phillip O., *et al.: Medical Parasitology*. New York: Appleton-Century-Crofts, 1963. Linear program.

Owen, S. G.: *Electrocardiography*. Boston, Mass.: Little, Brown & Co., 1966. Branching program. (Filmed version of program for use with the Grundytutor teaching machine is also available, see below.)

Owen, S. G.: *Principles of Electrocardiography*. Ashford, Middlesex, England: International Tutor Machines, Ltd. Branching program.

Physician's Liability for Battery, Negligence, and Acts of Others. Developed jointly by Educational Design, Inc., and Pfizer *Spectrum*, 1966. Linear program.

Primary Arterial Hypertension. Developed by Basic Systems, Inc. for A. A. G. P. and Merck Sharp and Dohme. Published serially in GP, July 1964-March 1965. Also obtainable directly from Merck Sharp and Dohme, West Point, Pa. Linear program.

Raymond, M. J., and Robertson, J.P.S.: *Programmed Series on Psychiatry*. Manchester, England: Geigy Pharmaceutical Co., 1965-66. Four volumes in six parts. Linear program.

Reinecke, R. D., and Herm, R. S.: *Refraction*. New York: Appleton-Century-Crofts, 1965. Linear program using a three dimensional viewer for frame presentation.

Reinecke, R. D., and Miller, David: *Strabismus: A Programmed Text*. New York: Appleton-Century-Crofts, 1966. Linear program.

Richardson, Fred MacD.: *The Physiology of Menstruation*. Philadelphia: The Pennsylvania Hospital, 1964. Linear program. Field test edition currently out of print.

Rondell, Paul: *Diffusion and Osmosis*. Ann Arbor: University of Michigan, 1963. Linear program. Also available in a Spanish edition translated by Luis Daufi, of the University of Barcelona School of Medicine.

Sackheim, George L.: *A Programmed Approach to the Circulatory System*. Champaign, Illinois: Stipes, 1963. Linear program.

Sidman, R. L., and Sidman, J.: *Neuroanatomy*. Boston: Little, Brown & Co., 1964. Linear program.

Sierra-Franco, M. H., and Krosnick, A.: *Diabetes Control: A Review Course*. New York: U. S. Industries, Inc., 1963. Branching program (for Auto-Tutor teaching machine).

Truelson, Stanley, D., Jr.: *How to Search the Medical Literature*. Rochester, New York: University of Rochester Medical Library, 1964. Linear program.

Urology. Developed jointly by Warner-Chilcott Laboratories and Basic Systems, Inc. New York: Warner-Chilcott Laboratories, 1965. Linear program.

Weller, John M., and Greene, James A., Jr.: *Examination of the Urine*. New York: Appleton-Century-Crofts, 1966. Linear program, includes color transparencies and slide viewer.

Wilds, P. L., and Zachert, V.: *Essentials of Gynecologic Oncology*. Augusta, Georgia: Medical College of Georgia, 1964. Linear program.

Wolf, A. V., and Crowder, N. A.: *An Introduction to Body Fluid Metabolism*. Baltimore: Williams & Wilkins Company, 1964. Branching program.

Articles on Para-Medical Programming

Bitzer, Marilyn: Self-directed inquiry in clinical nursing instruction by means of the PLATO simulated laboratory. University of Illinois Coordinated Science Laboratory Report R-184, 1963.
A comparative study of medical-surgical nursing instruction taught by means of a specially created computer-assisted program. Post-test results favored those students taught by the program and the teaching machine.

Carter, E. J., Moore, A. N., and Gregory, C. L.: Can teaching machines help in training employees? *J. Amer. Diet. Ass.* 44:271-276 (April) 1964.
A report on the controlled study of a program on hygiene and sanitation used with 68 unskilled food handlers. A significant increase in learning and retention was achieved by the program group.

Craytor, Josephine K., and Lysaught, Jerome P.: Programmed instruction in nursing education: A trial use. *Nursing Research*. 13:323-326 (Fall) 1964.
Report of a controlled study using programmed materials in radiation therapy for nursing students. 81 subjects participated. Effective and efficient learning results were achieved. Some evidence of reduced range in achievement was reported.

Feldman, Herman: Programmed instruction: What it is, how hospitals can use it. *The Modern Hospital*. 99:75-79 (October) 1962.
An orientation article for the hospital administrator on the use of programmed instruction.

Geis, George L., and Anderson, Maja C.: Programmed instruction in nursing education. *Nursing Outlook*. 11: (Part 1, August; Part 2, September) 1963.
A two-part paper describing fundamental aspects of programmed instruction and relating it to the concerns of nursing education.

Hector, Winifred E.: Making a programme. *Nursing Times*. 60: (June 5, 12, 19) 1964.

A series of articles suggesting a method for developing and constructing programs for use in nursing education.

Hinsvark, Inez G.: Programming procedural skills in the operating room. *Hospital Topics*. 41:55-58 (August) 1963.
Report of beginning efforts to program manual skills in nursing education.

Koehler, Margaret L.: Programmed instruction—potential uses in nursing. *Hospital Topics*. 41:48-50 (August) 1963.
An introductory discussion to a series of reports (see Hinsvark and Seedor) on programs utilized for nursing instruction.

MacDonald, Mary E. (ed.): *Programmed Instruction for Nursing*. Boston: Massachusetts League for Nursing, 1963.
Proceedings of the Institute on Programmed Instruction for Nursing held in November, 1963. Three papers plus excerpts from group discussions.

McDonald, Glen W., and Kaufman, Mildred B.: Teaching machines for patients with diabetes. *J. Amer. Diet. Ass.* 42:209-213 (March) 1963.
A report of an early experiment on the use of programs and devices for the self-education of patients.

Polony, Louis J.: Programmed instruction and automated education for hospitals and other medical personnel. *Hosp. Progr.* 46:83-87 (February) 1965.
An introductory article for the hospital administrator on the utilization of programmed materials.

Raine, N. L.: An experiment in programmed learning (Parts 1 and 2). *Nursing Times*. Vol. 62, #22, 23 (June) 1966.
A progress report on the first stages of planning and writing a program for nurses on disturbances of body fluid and electrolytes.

Seedor, Marie M.: Programmed instruction for a unit on asepsis. *Hospital Topics*. 41:50-5 (August) 1963.
Report on the development of a programmed unit for community college nursing students.

Self-teaching in the hospital. *Lancet*. 1:1055-56 (May) 1965.
A report and brief description of self-instructional developments for health education in the United States and Britain. Abbreviated discussion of early experimental results with suggestions for future applications.

Shindell, S.: Programmed instruction and its usefulness for the health professions. *Am. J. Pub. Health*. 54:982-990 (June) 1964.
A general discussion of the possibilities for improving health profession teaching through an enlargement of self-instructional approaches. Gives a discursive view of the developing field of programmed instruction in the health professions.

Skiff, Anna W.: Programmed instruction and patient teaching. *Amer. J. Public Health*. 55:409-415 (March) 1965.

A discussion of results obtained in the use of self-instructional materials for patient management of health problems.

Spiegel, Allen D.: Patient and physician education. *Medical Care* 3:46-51 (January-March) 1965.
Further analysis of the use of programs for both physician and patient on aspects of diabetes management.

Spiegel, Allen D.: The teaching machine. *Postgrad. Med.* 39:4:A84-A90 (April) 1966.
An analysis of reactions and results in the use of a self-instructional program designed for practitioners.

Programmed Units in Para-Medical Fields

Amebiasis: Laboratory Diagnosis. (Introduction and three parts.) Atlanta, Georgia: USPHS Communicable Disease Center, 1964. (PHS Publication #1187). Linear, mathetics program.

Anderson, Maja C.: *Basic Nursing Techniques.* (Vol. II of a programmed course in nursing fundamentals.) Philadelphia: W. B. Saunders Co., 1968. Linear program. (In press)

Anderson, Maja C.: *Basic Patient Care.* (Vol. I of a programmed course in nursing fundamentals.) Philadelphia: W. B. Saunders Co., 1965. Linear program.

Anderson, Ruth M., and Silver, Eva: *Ward management for quality patient care.* American Journal of Nursing. 66:567-590 (March) 1966. Linear program.

Anthony, Catherine Parker: *Basic Concepts of Anatomy and Physiology.* St. Louis: C. V. Mosby Co., 1966.
Linear programmed manual for nursing students.

Anti-Inflammatory Agents. New York: Basic Systems, Inc., 1964.
Linear program for pharmacists, consisting of three units: inflammation, inflammatory diseases, and current anti-inflammatory therapy.

Basic Concepts of Human Anatomy and Physiology. Developed jointly by Bolt, Beranek, and Newman and Wyeth Laboratories. Philadelphia: Wyeth Laboratories, 1964.
Linear program consisting of nine units in five volumes.

Biologicals and Immunology. New York: Basic Systems, Inc., 1964.
Linear program for pharmacists.

Brooks, Stewart M.: *Basic Chemistry: A Programmed Presentation.* St. Louis: C. V. Mosby Co., 1966.
Linear program for nursing students.

Carter, Evelyn, and Moore, Aimee: *Food Sanitation.* New York: U. S. Industries, Inc., 1964.
Branching program for food handlers and nonprofessional employees.

Chemistry of the Nervous System. New York: Basic Systems, Inc., 1965.
Linear program for pharmacists.

Cherescavich, Gertrude, and Fagen, Claire. *Anxiety Recognition and Intervention.* Developed with Basic Systems, Inc. *American Journal of Nursing.* 65:9:129-152 (September) 1965.
Linear program for nurses.
Clinical Oral Pathology (Revision). Ashford, Middlesex, England: International Tutor Machines Ltd., 1966.
Branching program for dentistry students.
Clinical Pharmacology. New York: Basic Systems, Inc., 1965.
Linear program for pharmacists.
Closed Drainage of the Chest: A Programmed Course for Nurses. Washington, D. C.: U. S. Department of Health, Education, and Welfare, Public Health Service Publication No. 1337, 1965.
Linear program for nurses.
Dermatology. New York: Basic Systems, Inc., 1965.
Linear program for pharmacists, consisting of three units: the skin, anatomy and physiology; skin diseases, and skin therapy.
Diabetic Therapy. New York: Basic Systems, Inc., 1965.
Linear program for pharmacists.
Diuretics and Antihypertensive Agents. New York: Basic Systems, Inc., 1964.
Linear program for pharmacists, consisting of five units: the circulatory system and blood pressure control; hypertension and antihypertensive agents; electrolyte balance and diffusion of body fluids; kidney structure and function; and diuretics.
Elements of Corticosteroid Pharmacology. New York: Basic Systems, Inc., 1964.
Linear program for pharmacists, consisting of four units: introduction to the corticosteroids; the effect of corticosteroids on metabolism; disorders of the adrenal cortex; and corticosteroid therapy.
Female Endocrinology: The Sex Hormones. New York: Basic Systems, Inc., 1964.
Linear program for pharmacists.
The Female Reproductive System. New York: Basic Systems, Inc., 1964.
Linear program for pharmacists.

Ferster, Charles: *Arithmetic for Nurses.* New York: Springer, 1965.
Linear program for nurses and technicians.

Frye, Charles, Paulson, Casper, and Spitz, Harold: *Dental Anatomy: A Self-Instructional Program.* Portland, Ore.: Oregon State System of Higher Education, 1965.
A modified branching-linear program for dentists, oral surgeons, and others involved in dental anatomy.
Fungus Diseases. New York: Basic Systems, Inc., 1965.
Linear program for pharmacists.
General Relationship Development Program. Atlanta: Human Development Institute.
Linear program designed for use by two individuals working as a pair;

for use by nurses or others seeking to improve interpersonal effectiveness.
Glucose Metabolism and Diabetes. New York: Basic Systems, Inc., 1965.
Linear program for pharmacists.

Goodell, Helen, and Rhymes, Julina P.: *Pain: Part 1, Basic Concepts and Assessment.* American Journal of Nursing. 66:1085-1108 (May) 1966. Linear program.

Harrison, James D., and Podshadley, Arlon G.: *Cavity Preparation and Impression Taking.* St. Louis, Mo.: C. V. Mosby Co., 1965.
Teaching program for dental students.

Hart, Laura K.: *The Arithmetic of Dosages and Solutions.* St. Louis, Mo.: C. V. Mosby, Inc., 1965. Linear program for student nurses.

Hector, Winifred: *Food for the Diabetic.* London, England: William Heinemann Ltd., 1965.
Branching program for nurses.

Hector, Winifred: *Measuring Insulin.* Bristol, England: Teaching Systems Ltd., 1966.
Linear program for student nurses.

Hector, Winifred: *Red Blood Cells.* Bristol, England: Teaching Systems Ltd., 1966.
Branching program for student nurses.
Hypotension and Shock. New York: Basic Systems, Inc., 1964.
Linear program for pharmacists.
Insecticide Formulation. Atlanta, Georgia: USPHS Communicable Disease Center, 1965.
Linear, mathetics program for technicians and laboratory personnel.
Introduction to Dental Public Health. Public Health Service Publication No. 1134. Washington, D. C.: U. S. Department of Health, Education and Welfare. Linear program.
Jet Injector Operation, Model K3. Atlanta, Georgia: USPHS Communicable Disease Center, 1965. Linear, mathetics program.

Keane, Claire, and Fletcher, Sybil: *Drugs and Solutions: A Programmed Introduction for Nurses.* Philadelphia: W. B. Saunders, 1965. Linear program for nurses.

Krueger, Elizabeth A.: *The Hypodermic Injection: A Programmed Unit.* New York: Teachers College Press, 1966.
Linear program for nurses. (Also available from J. B. Lippincott Co., Philadelphia, Pa.)

Lipsey, Sally: *Mathematics for Nursing Science: A Programmed Review.* New York: John Wiley & Sons, 1965.
Linear program for nurses.

Malcolm, Barbara, and Bielski, Mary: *Recognizing Signs of Internal Hemorrhage.* Developed with Basic Systems, Inc. *American Journal of*

Nursing. 65:12:119-138 (December) 1965.
Linear program for nurses.

Malcolm, Barbara, and Glor, Beverly: *Correcting Common Errors in Blood Pressure Measurement.* Developed with Basic Systems, Inc. *American Journal of Nursing.* 65:10:133-164 (October) 1965.
Linear program for nurses.

Malcolm, Barbara, and Miller, Marjorie: *Intravenous Infusion of Vasopressors.* Developed with Basic Systems, Inc. *American Journal of Nursing.* 65:11:129-152 (November) 1965.
Linear program for nurses.

Medical Physiology. Wilmette, Illinois: Encyclopedia Britannica Press, 1965.
Linear program for the adult lay reader.
Mental Illness. New York: Basic Systems, Inc., 1964.
Linear program for pharmacists.
Microbiology and Antibiotics. New York: Basic Systems, Inc., 1964.
Linear program for pharmacists, consisting of two units: microbiology; and antibiotics.
The Nervous System. New York: Basic Systems, Inc., 1964.
Linear program for pharmacists.
Nutrition. Middlesex, England: Educational Systems Ltd., 1966.
Mixed program (Linear and Branching) for student nurses. Designed for use on a teaching machine.

O'Brien, William, and Ryge, Gunnar: *Dental Materials: A Programmed Review of Selected Topics.* Philadelphia: W. B. Saunders, 1965.
Linear program for dental students.

Plym, Alberta, and Aikawa, J.: *Programmed Instruction in Medical Technology.* Denver: The University of Colorado Medical Center, Central Laboratory, 1965.
Linear programs for medical students and technologists, consisting of six units: acidosis and alkalosis, diagnostic aids in thyroid disorders, instrumentation, evaluation of laboratory data, potassium metabolism, and basic statistics.
Programmed Instruction in the use of ICDA. Ann Arbor, Michigan: Commission on Professional & Hospital Activities, Inc., 1963.
Linear program for indexing Hospital records by disease and operations.
Programmed Instruction—Respiratory Tract Aspiration. New York, N. Y.: American Journal of Nursing, 1966.
Linear program for nurses.
Psychopharmacology. New York: Basic Systems, Inc., 1964.
Linear program for pharmacists.

Rains, A. J. Harding, Carpenter, Mary F., and Goodman, Richard (eds.): *The Mechanism of Respiration and Closed Drainage of the Pleural Cavity.* London, England: English Universities Press Ltd., 1966.
Two teaching programmes for nurses.

Rehabilitative Aspects of Nursing: A Programmed Instruction Series.
New York: National League for Nursing, 1966.
Linear program for nurses.
Renal Physiology and Basic Urology. New York: Basic Systems, Inc.,
1964.
Linear program for pharmacists.

Sackheim, G. I., and Robins, L.: *Programmed Mathematics for Nurses.*
New York: Macmillan, 1964. Linear program.

Saxton, Dolores F., and Walter, John F.: *Programmed Instruction in
Arithmetic, Dosages, and Solutions.* St. Louis: C. V. Mosby Co., 1966.
Linear programmed text-workbook for nurses.

Seedor, Marie M.: *Aids to Diagnosis: A Programmed Unit in Fundamentals of Nursing.* New York: Teachers College, Columbia University,
1964. Branching program.

Seedor, Marie M.: *Inhalation Therapy: A Programmed Unit in Fundamentals of Nursing.* New York: Teachers College, Columbia University, 1965. Branching program.

Seedor, Marie M.: *Introduction to Asepsis: A Programmed Unit in
Fundamentals of Nursing.* New York: Teachers College, Columbia
University, 1963. Branching program.

Seedor, Marie M.: *Therapy with Oxygen and Other Gases: A Pro-
grammed 'Unit in Fundamentals of Nursing.* New York: Teachers Col-
lege, Columbia University, 1967.
Branching program for basic training in inhalation therapy.
Selected Medical Terminology: A Self-Instruction Lesson Manual. New
York: The United Hospital Fund of New York and Lenox Hill Hospi-
tal, 1963. (Distributed by Teco Instruction, Inc., 3236 N. E. 12th Ave.,
Ft. Lauderdale, Florida.)
Modified linear program for nurses and technicians.
The Sex Hormones. New York: Basic Systems, Inc., 1964.
Linear program for pharmacists.

Smith, G. L., and Davis, P. E.: *Medical Terminology.* New York: John
Wiley & Sons, 1963.
Linear program for technicians and medical secretaries; also has been
used with nurses.
Sterilisation Techniques. Middlesex, England: Educational Systems
Ltd., 1966. Designed for use on a Teaching Machine.
Mixed program (Linear and Branching) for student nurses.
Taking Care of Diabetes. New York: U. S. Industries, Inc., 1964.
Branching program for patients.
*Temperature, Pulse, and Respiration Measurement: A Programmed
Notebook for Nursing Assistants.* Bethesda, Md.: U. S. Department of
Health, Education, and Welfare, Public Health Service Publication No.
1456, 1966.
Linear program consisting of five parts.

Wilcox, Jane: *Blood Pressure Measurement: A Programmed Notebook for Nurses.* Washington, D. C.: U. S. Department of Health, Education and Welfare, Public Health Service, Publication No. 1191, 1964. Modified linear program for nurses.

General Health Programs

The following units were designed for junior high school learners, but they may have applications in specific need areas such as review, nonprofessional training, etc.:

Bolden, LeRoy, Jr.: *Safety.* Palo Alto: Behavioral Research Laboratory, 1964.
Linear text with teacher's manual and test booklet.

Igel, B. Haller: *Body Structure and Function.* Palo Alto: Behavioral Research Laboratory, 1966.
Linear text with teacher's manual and test booklet.

Igel, B. Haller: *First Aid.* Palo Alto: Behavioral Research Laboratory, 1964.
Linear text with teacher's manual and test booklet.

Igel, B. Haller: *Personal Health.* Palo Alto: Behavioral Research Laboratory, 1966.
Linear text with teacher's manual and test booklet.

Igel, B. Haller: *Prevention of Communicable Disease.* Palo Alto: Behavioral Research Laboratory, 1965.
Linear text with teacher's manual and test booklet.

Igel, B. Haller, and Calloway, Dorris H.: *Nutrition.* Palo Alto: Behavioral Research Laboratory, 1964.
Linear text with teacher's manual and test booklet.

Cumulative Index

---

*NOTE: References in *italics* are found in the first proceedings, PROGRAMMED INSTRUCTION IN MEDICAL EDUCATION;
References in **bold face** are found in this volume.